Essential Ophthalmol

Essential Ophthalmology

Hector Bryson Chawla

MB ChB(St.And), DO(Lond), DRCOG(Lond), FRCS(Edin)

Consultant Ophthalmic Surgeon, Royal Infirmary, Edinburgh; Examiner, Royal College of Surgeons, Edinburgh, and Royal College of Physicians and Surgeons, Glasgow

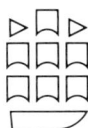

CHURCHILL LIVINGSTONE
EDINBURGH LONDON MELBOURNE AND NEW YORK 1981

CHURCHILL LIVINGSTONE
Medical Division of Longman Group Limited

Distributed in the United States of America by
Churchill Livingstone Inc., 1560 Broadway, New York,
N.Y. 10036, and by associated companies, branches and
representatives throughout the world.

First edition 1981
  Reprinted 1983

ISBN 0 443 021716

British Library Cataloguing in Publication Data
Chawla, Hector Bryson
Essential Ophthalmology.
1. Ophthalmology
617.7   RE46   80–41652

**Printed in Hong Kong by
Wilture Printing Co. Ltd.**

Preface

This book appeals to reason and not to memory. It presents the eye as an arrangement of standard tissues that happen to be transparent in places—an organ with a limited number of responses to a limitless number of insults and only a few symptoms to describe them with.

From this concept of limited response flows understanding. Each ocular structure has its own individual requirement for continued health. Suspend these requirements and we have a malfunction. Vary the cause of this suspension and we generally have the same malfunction.

For example, the conjunctiva may become inflamed because of tear deficiency, or because of infection, or because an eyelid has fallen away from the globe. But all these are still recognisable as conjunctivitis, and all three can be recognised separately in their own right if the eye is examined in the same way every time.

Now this is not just another medical discipline acquired through weary hours of self denial. It is a brief elementary ritual that can be mastered in as short a time as it takes to perform it. And in common with similar rituals for other systems it will tell us not only what is wrong, but also what is not wrong—often the more important thing to be told.

The evolving patterns of these things that go wrong and their management follow logically from an uncomplicated understanding of the normal eye and of general pathology. Emphasis has been given to their early identification before they have developed beyond the scope of treatment into medical curiosities.

I hope this text fills a gap in the ophthalmic literature. The material has been balanced between the academic and the practical. The former might bring examination candidates to terms with the subject, and to the composition of their lonely essays. The latter might bring solace to those faced with even more lonely decisions; it might also prevent them from making the same mistake a thousand times and calling it experience.

Edinburgh, 1981   H. B. C.

Acknowledgements

My grateful thanks are due to my secretary, Mrs Ena Vaughan, who cheerfully kept providing one final manuscript after another; to Mr Ian Lennox of the Medical Illustration Service, Edinburgh University, whose illustrations fill the gaps where words alone are not enough; to Dr Clifford Mawdsley, Consultant Neurologist, Royal Infirmary, Edinburgh, for his encouraging and constructive appraisal of the script; to Dr George Beveridge, Consultant Dermatologist, Royal Infirmary, Edinburgh, for his advice on skin deseases and the eye; and to Sutton Siebert Publications with whom I have published some of the ideas developed in this book. I am however most indebted to my colleague, Dr Lorna Young, who unearthed errors of fact, taste and reason in a manuscript that I had long thought perfect.

Contents

1

The common tissues that make up the eye

The whole point of the eye is to see. It achieves this by transmitting light through a series of transparent structures to a sensitive film—the retina—which lines its posterior cavity. Its position, shape, formation and behaviour are all subordinate to this end.

At first glance it would seem that very special tissues are necessary to perform this marvel and, at an emotional level, indeed they are. However, anatomy knows no emotion, and these tissues are to be found elsewhere in the body. Even the transparent ones, although specific to the eye, have features in common with their opaque fellows. The onslaught of disease makes these similarities even more marked.

Each eye points forwards from a bony cavity in the skull, called the orbit (Fig. 1). It is protected in front by the eyelashes, commonly known as hair in other circumstances, and a regular prey to eager beauticians.

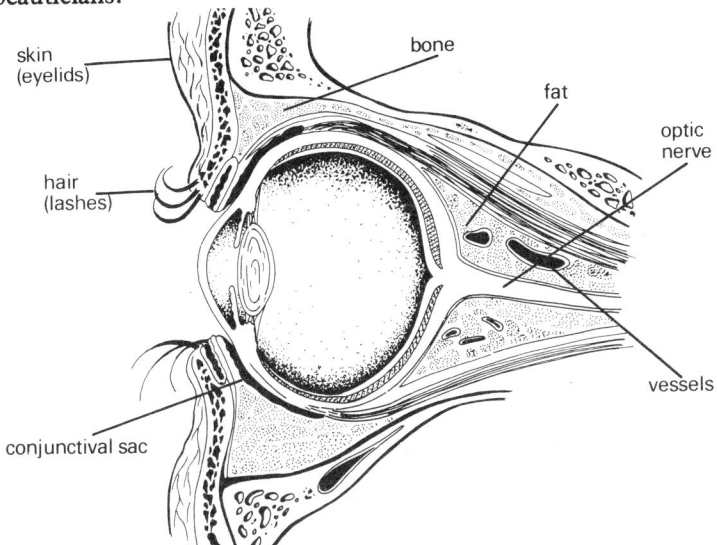

Fig. 1 An assembly of commonplace tissues

The eyelids, of normal skin, whose shape is maintained by a fibrous plate, are opened and shut by muscles. They are lined on their deep surface by a 'synovial' membrane, called the conjunctiva, that folds backwards on to the globe as a sac which then comes forwards again to blend with the clear window at the front of the eye—the cornea (Fig. 2).

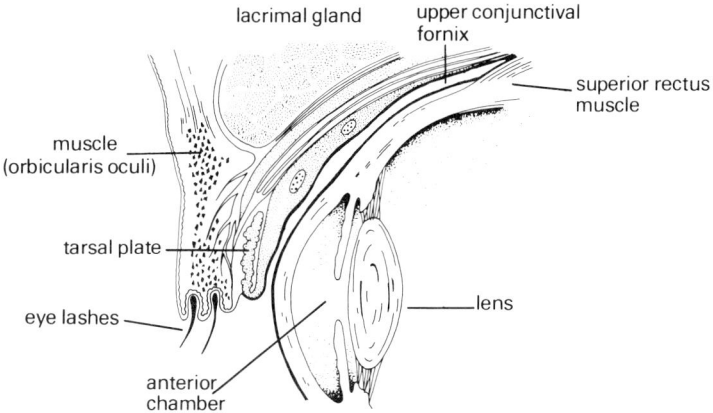

Fig. 2 The tear moist alliance between the eyelids, the conjunctiva and the cornea

This membrane is kept moist by a salty solution of tears, flowing from the lacrimal gland. This is not unlike a salivary gland and sits above the eye behind the conjunctival sac.

Although well known as demonstrations of sorrow, emotion, frustration, and blackmail, tears have a more prosaic though no less important function related to their role as a blood substitute for the cornea. Superflous tears normally drain away through little holes in the eyelids and along minute canals to collect in a tear sac, whence they flow along another duct into the nose.

The outer coat of the globe (the sclera) is like the ball of a joint, which moves in a socket of muscle, bone and eyelids (Fig. 3). It is formed of collagen fibres, and is heir to the same diseases as suffered by collagen elsewhere.

Its transparent anterior portion, the cornea, begins the process of bending transmitted light towards a point focus on the retina (Fig. 4).

The middle coat of the eye is a mixture of blood vessels, pigment cells and muscle, woven together by connective tissue. It is visible in front as the iris, where its dappled shades have given rise to much languid poetry and not a few rash decisions. The hole in the centre of the iris is called the pupil. The pupil constricts to protect the retina

conjunctival
'synovial' membrane

conjunctiva
stretched

conjunctiva
flung
into
folds

muscle relaxed

muscle
contracted

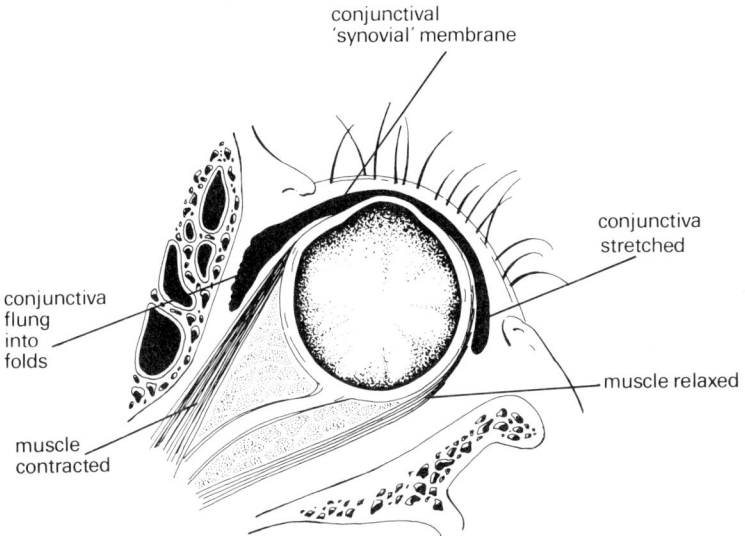

Fig. 3 The eye moving like a ball and socket joint

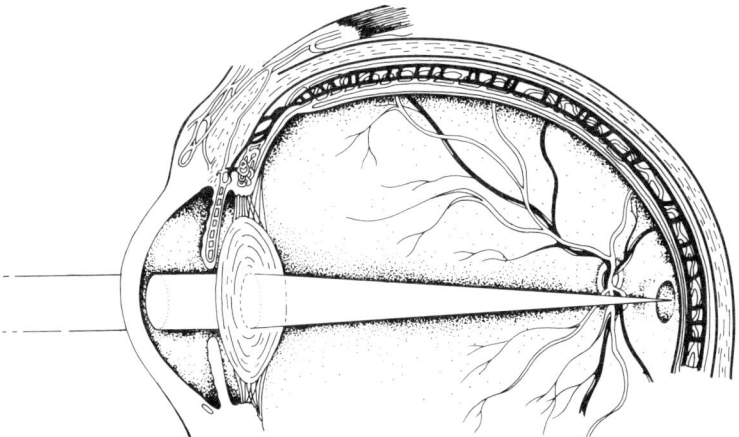

Fig. 4 A cone of light brought to a point focus at the macula by the cornea and the lens

from excess light, and dilates to allow the eye to make the best use of what light might be available (Fig. 5).

The iris merges backwards into the ciliary body, the source of the aqueous fluid which continually circulates through the pupil en route to the angle of the anterior chamber (Fig. 6), whence it is drained from the eye by veins in the sclera.

The ciliary body continues backwards now as the choroid, which

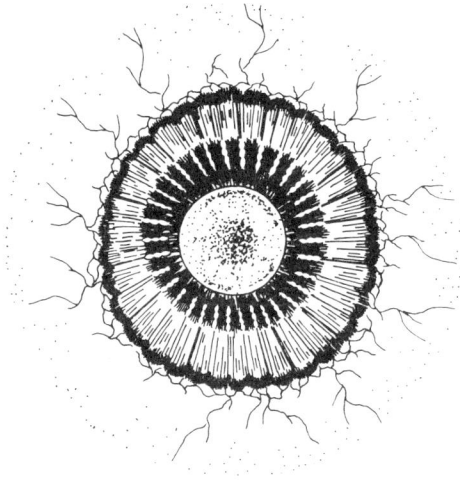

Fig. 5 The iris and pupil seen through the cornea and the fine network of vessels encircling the corneo-scleral limbus and seen better if seen closer with a small convex lens (+ lens)

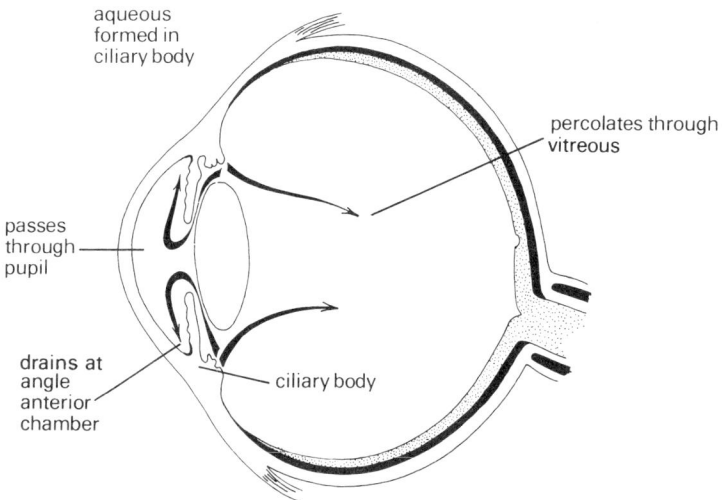

aqueous
formed in
ciliary body

percolates through
vitreous

passes
through
pupil

drains at
angle
anterior
chamber

ciliary body

Fig. 6 The aqueous circulation
Unsuspected when circulating well; unsuspected when not circulating well

feeds the retina and is the basis of that familiar red glow noted so gratefully in the case records after a cataract extraction.

Collectively the three are called the uveal tract, from their fancied and happily rare resemblance to a succulent Burgundy grape, when disease has thinned the covering sclera into bulging translucency.

The inner coat is the retina—a continuation forwards of the optic nerve, and both are part of the brain. Like all special tissues it has reached such a pinnacle of refinement that it has totally lost the ability to reproduce itself. The retina in fact consists of two distinct layers—an outer pigment layer and an inner neural layer. These merge at the anterior limit of the functioning retina—the ora serrata—a landmark more familiar in name than position. These fused layers continue forwards to line the deep surface of the ciliary body and of the iris.

Within the globe there are now two further transparent structures. Dangling from the ciliary body is the lens which, in response to a muscle attached also to the ciliary body (the ciliary muscle) can modify the focus of the transmitted light.

Behind the lens the posterior cavity of the eye is filled with vitreous gel—sometimes referred to by the quainter term of vitreous humour. Somewhat of the consistency of waterglass, it lies in contact with the optic nerve head, the retina, part of the ciliary body and the lens (Fig. 7).

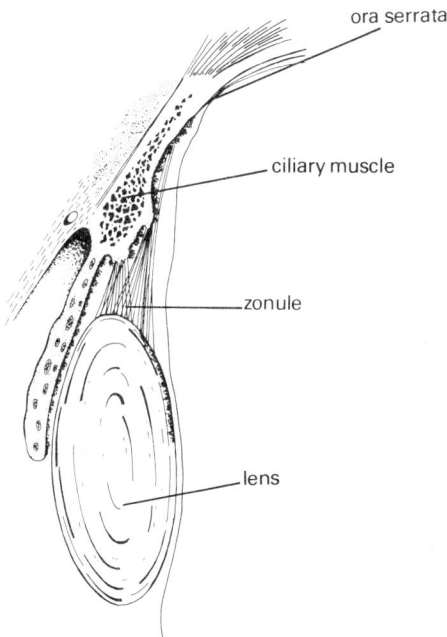

Fig. 7 The anterior relations of the vitreous gel and its adherence to the retina at the ora serrata

So much for the inside of the eye. The tissues on the outside are concerned with eye movements, pain sensation and shock absorption. Each eye is moved by six muscles, which can be regarded as voluntary although there is, however, an involuntary component to their action (Fig. 8). Of course, there are two eyes and each gazes upon the world from a different viewpoint. The brain fuses these different flat views into one view in depth. We call this *binocular vision*.

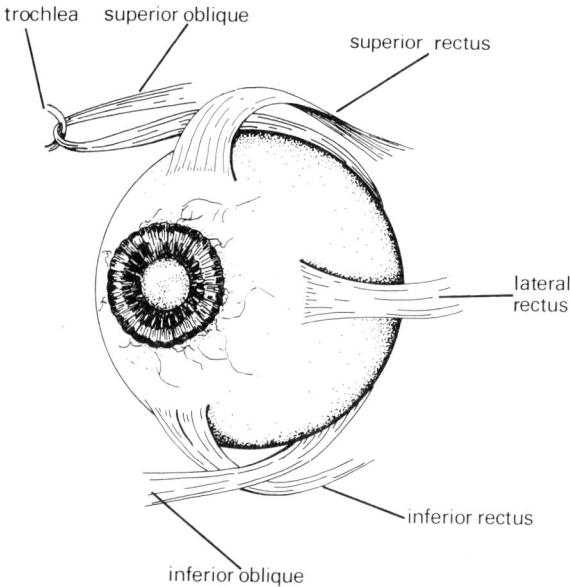

Fig. 8 The extra ocular muscles of the left eye

The remaining space in the orbital cavity is filled with arteries, veins, cranial nerves and fat.

The organ of mystery must now be emerging prosaically as just another collection of familiar tissues—curious perhaps in its shape, worrying in the sum of its parts, but totally commonplace when each part is taken in isolation.

THE TRANSPARENT TISSUES

In order to see, the eye has to be transparent in places—its one unique quality. Any slight independence in its normal behaviour pivots around that one fact.

The three transparent structures are the cornea, the lens and the vitreous. The retinal layers nearest to the light are also transparent, but short of remarking upon that we need examine it no further.

There is also the aqueous humour which fills the anterior chamber and any other gaps within the ocular cavity, and this is also clear like so many other water-based liquids.

The common factor in transparency is an absence of blood vessels, because these of course are not transparent. However, as the structures are living tissues they require a blood substitute to provide nutrition, oxygen and a waste disposal system.

The specialist tissues throughout the body, although separate in their function, unite in their preference for the complex over the simple. However, such complexity flourishes only when circumstances are favourable, and disease processes tend to infiltrate their state of patrician refinement with common connective tissue— sometimes to the point of total replacement.

The cornea

The cornea (Fig. 9) transmits light and because of its convexity, focuses light as well. Its well-being starts with snugly fitting eyelids that blink reflexly to remove unwanted foreign bodies and to coat its surface with a smooth film of tears, making the cornea glistening as any quality refracting surface should. Anything that separates the lids from the cornea—for example a facial nerve palsy—puts this smooth surface in danger of replacement by keratinised epithelium. This is excellent as a protective layer, but not so good when it comes to seeing.

With a blood supply confined to its margins, the cornea relies on tears to act as a blood substitute for its anterior epithelial layer. An occasional proof of this need is the epithelial clouding that flourishes deep to a negligently over-worn contact lens.

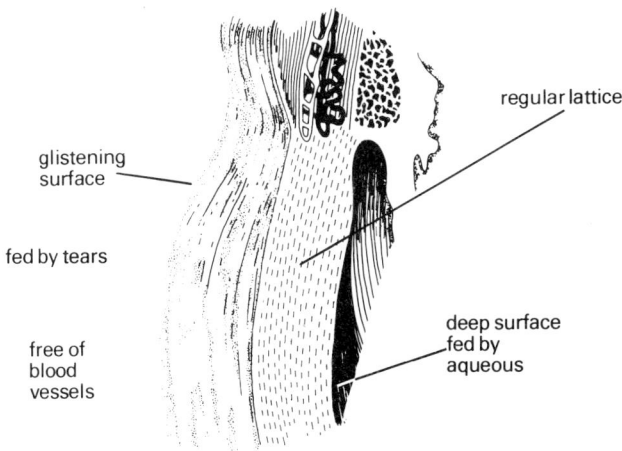

glistening
surface

regular lattice

fed by tears

deep surface
fed by
aqueous

free of
blood
vessels

Fig. 9 How the cornea stays clear

The corneal stroma

As the forward continuation of the sclera, the cornea of course plays its part in maintaining the spherical shape of the eyeball and in protecting its contents. Its collagen fibres, though no different from those of the sclera in form, are rather different in their arrangement. This actual arrangement has taxed the ingenuity of theorists, who have still not convincingly explained the corneal transparency. However it is alleged that these fibres lie in a two-dimensional lattice just less than a wavelength of light apart. By some subtle and as yet unexplained mechanism, light passes through where, in some other arrangement, it might not (Fig. 10). This hypothesis is borne out clinically by the scar formation—as opaque as any part of the sclera—that follows any disturbance of the corneal stroma.

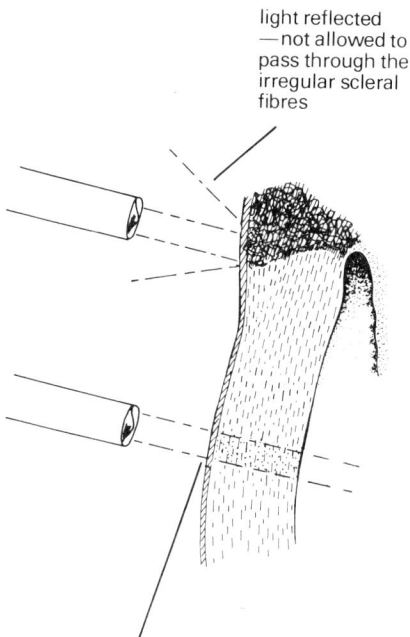

light reflected —not allowed to pass through the irregular scleral fibres

Fig. 10 Light is transmitted only through a regular corneal lattice

Two membranes mark the limits of the stroma. Its anterior suface is separated from the anterior epithelial layer by Bowman's Membrane, penetration of which will always result in a scar.

Its deep concave surface is lined by Descemet's Membrane, which separates the stroma from the deep cellular endothelial layer.

This endothelial layer plays a vital part in the maintenance of corneal clarity. It continually withdraws water from the corneal stroma to keep it in a state of semi-hydration. Any disturbance of this layer, for example the deposition of inflammatory debris on the endothelium, will block this outflow of water with resultant corneal oedema (Fig. 11). The aqueous humour acts as the blood substitute of this deep corneal surface.

The cornea thus consists of five layers—two cellular, two membranous and one collagenous.

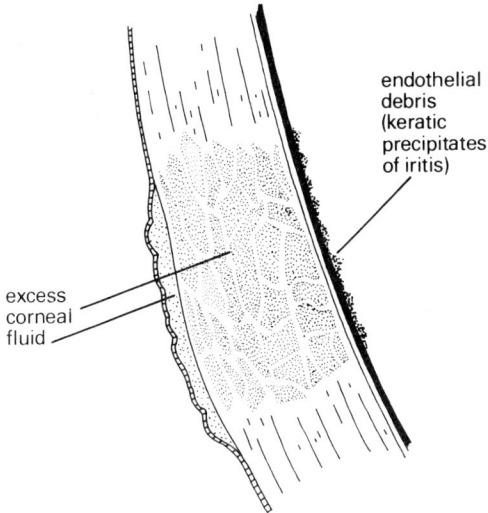

Fig. 11 Corneal oedema
Iritic debris interfering with the suction mechanism of the endothelium

The lens
This structure is layered like an onion but shaped like a lentil and held so by a cellular capsule from which its 'onion fibres' are derived.

The ciliary body from which it is suspended contains a muscle stretching fore and aft from the sclero-corneal junction. This is the muscle of accommodation, which on contraction allows the lens to become more convex to keep the eye in focus for near objects. This near point of focus recedes with age because the hardening lens responds less and less to the muscle of accommodation. It is left to parents to make this tetchy discovery when children, comfortably in focus six inches from the television screen, thrust baubles for attention rather closer to the nose than an ageing near point can cope with.

The blood substitute of the lens is the aqueous humour and any insult, whether an alteration in the composition of the aqueous or damage to the lens capsule, brings with it the risk of clouding. Whatever the cause, this loss of transparency can be called cataract, but preferably not within earshot of patients, who all go in mortal dread of the name.

The vitreous humour

This is possibly the most inert tissue of the body, making the standard tendon seem almost lively by comparison. A whorl of fine collagenous fibrils separated by globules of hyaluronic acid gel, it fills the cavity of the eye behind the lens. Its attachments in health are to the optic nerve and the ora serrata. The aqueous fluid drifting through serves its languid metabolic functions. Any opacities resulting from disease clear away with equal languor, if they do so at all.

The aqueous humour

It is critical to grasp the normal behaviour of this fluid, for the eye depends upon it for the maintenance of its health and the maintenance of its shape. What is more, many eye disorders bring influence to bear upon its circulation. It is here that diseases with multiple causation will rotate around a single pathological axis.

It is secreted in the ciliary body by those fused layers of cells that continue forwards from the retina. It flows through the pupil to fill the anterior chamber, where it feeds the lens and the deep surface of the cornea before filtering out of the eye through the angle of the anterior chamber (see Fig. 6).

The normal eye can be thought of as a soft walled sphere full of liquid, that forms within and flows out at an equal rate. This simple circulation of aqueous humour lies at the very core of the eye's existence.

Its pathological behaviour is equally simple. If its secretion ceases the eye will collapse. Disturbance of its contents can disturb the clear tissues in the globe dependent upon it. Blockage of its circulation at any point from its source in the ciliary body to the drainage angle will raise the pressure of the eyeball. This raised pressure is called glaucoma, and its qualifying name will vary depending on the exciting cause. When no cause is known, we call it primary glaucoma, or give our ignorance a scientific ring with the Latin alternative of *glaucoma simplex*.

SUMMARY

It must now be evident that the eye and its supporting structures have infinitely more in common with the rest of the body than is customarily supposed. All but three of the tissues are duplicated elsewhere. These three tissues share transparency as their common factor.

They achieve this quality by their internal arrangement, their shape and their dependence upon blood substitutes. When defeated by disease processes, they are prepared to change their unique privileges in return for a simple survival. Where once they played a rarified role, bathed in tears or aqueous, they descend to accept the infiltration of blood vessels rather than die. The price they pay, of course, is the loss of their special qualities. They are rather like a putting surface taken over by weeds—recognisable as grass but not as a green fit for displays of virtuosity.

As for the aqueous, this is perhaps the most misunderstood of all the intra-ocular contents. Most people have heard something about it, but cannot remember what they have heard and, if they do, cannot believe that that's all there is to it.

Now there may be some dispute over its exact mode of production, a mild academic wrangle over its precise composition, a confrontation of authorities over its mechanism of drainage. However, the clinical facts are beyond question. It is a blood substitute, it maintains the shape of the globe, and it circulates. If the eye goes wrong we must assume that the aqueous is involved somehow until we prove that it is not. A knowledge of these simple facts takes the management of ocular disorders from the realms of hope into the realms of scientific expectation.

2

How the eye sees and why it sometimes needs help

NORMAL VISION

The normal eye possesses two distinct visual faculties—central vision and field of vision.

Central vision

This talent is the preserve of a tiny area of retina lying in the posterior pole of the eye called the macula. Although tiny, the area is highly refined, permitting that precise distinction between almost similar details upon which so much of our daily life depends. This may range from reading a line of print to reading a number plate at a distance that might satisfy the licensing authorities. It also allows us to recognise the colour of the car attached to the number plate (Fig. 12). Just how tiny can be judged by trying to read adjacent words on a page of print whilst maintaining fixation on one of them.

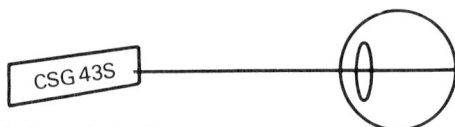

Fig. 12 Central vision—in the distance

It is the one kind of vision that everybody knows about. When something goes wrong with the central vision people are quick to complain. They make the mistake of thinking it the only kind of vision. They endow it with qualities that belong to another kind of vision altogether—field of vision (Fig. 13).

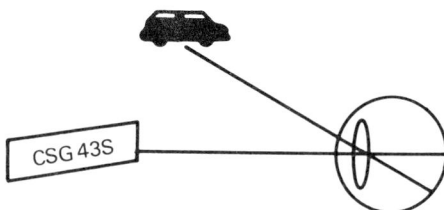

Fig. 13 Central vision and field of vision—in the distance

Field of vision

While any disturbance of the centre will produce a stream of patients wondering if the time has come to discard their grandmother's glasses, large areas of the visual field can disappear unnoticed. Yet this self effacing attribute is the more important one. We neglect it at our peril.

Served by the extra-macular retina, it depends on receptor cells called rods which, although useless for the recognition of colour, have the quality of increased sensitivity in the dark.

Each eye has a visual field shaped rather like a pear lying on its side, the stalk end pointing nasally, the bulbous end pointing temporally. With both eyes open there is clearly an overlap of these fields—circular in shape. This is called the binocular field (Fig. 14). Each eye,

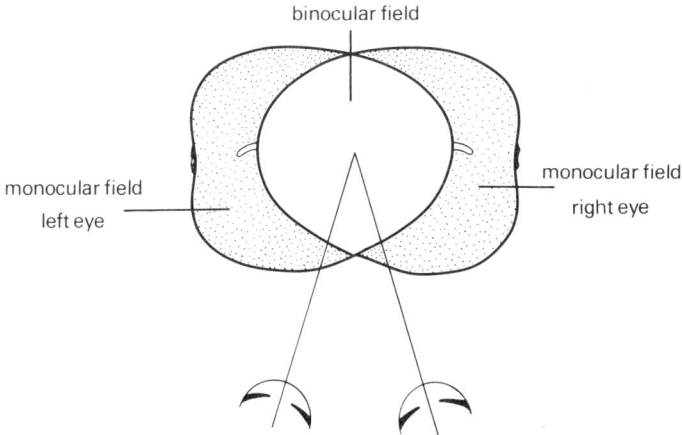

binocular field

monocular field
left eye

monocular field
right eye

Fig. 14 What the eyes can see together and what they see separately

however, retains a certain degree of independence, for the bulbous end of the pear on the temporal side provides a crescent of vision that belongs to that eye alone. This fact can be demonstrated by maintaining fixation with the central vision on some immobile distant object whilst covering each eye alternately.

With an intact pathway running from the macula to the occipital cortex, it would be reasonable to imagine that normal central vision would exist automatically. Unfortunately, as far as central vision is concerned, health alone is not enough, for central vision is not a birthright. An intact pathway will not allow normal vision to develop if circumstances for this development are unfavourable. A squinting eye is an example of such unfavourable circumstances.

There is some controversy about when it is too late to develop central vision. Some authorities claim success in establishing it up to eight years, others would limit it to five, while others still suggest that, unless the pathway has been opened for use by three months, it will never be open at all. In practical terms we have a diminishing opportunity up to the age of five to persuade the central vision to develop.

The peripheral retina collects impressions of our surroundings that become less rough the nearer these impressions approach the sensitive macula. Factors judged to be of interest by the peripheral retina and by the brain, depending on experience, taste, sex and youth, are selected for the privilege of a macular view, and if the macular interest strays then this peripheral retina edges it back on to fixation.

Quite disturbingly large areas of the field can be lost, and patients become concerned only when the loss creeps close enough to affect the macula, when they declare with some urgency and conviction that they have suddenly gone blind. Just because people can still see is no guarantee that they will continue to, for normal central vision is a valueless index of ocular health. Yet it is the only index in general use. Chronic glaucoma, an insidious disease of the elderly, may quietly remove most of the visual field, whilst its victims are deciding that next year will be time enough to replace their disintegrating spectacles.

THE RETINA

This first appears in the embryo as a small balloon on a stalk derived from the brain. The anterior half dimples, then dimples a little more and sinks into the cavity of the balloon, forming two layers. The inner layer becomes the neural retina. The outer layer becomes the pigment retina. These unite at their anterior limit—the ora serrata (Fig. 15).

As part of the brain the neural retina has an enormously complicated arrangement. However, its complications can be reduced to light receptors adjacent to the pigment retina, which then connect through a series of cells, finally ending as the nerve fibres of the innermost retinal layer. These fibres sweep from all areas of the retina, leaving the eye through the optic nerve head, also described as the optic disc or the papilla.

These light receptors contain an aldehyde of vitamin A linked with a protein molecule, and it is the realignment of these molecules in response to light that gives rise to visual perception.

Cones

Such receptors abound in the macula where, as well as providing visual precision, they also distinguish one colour from the next.

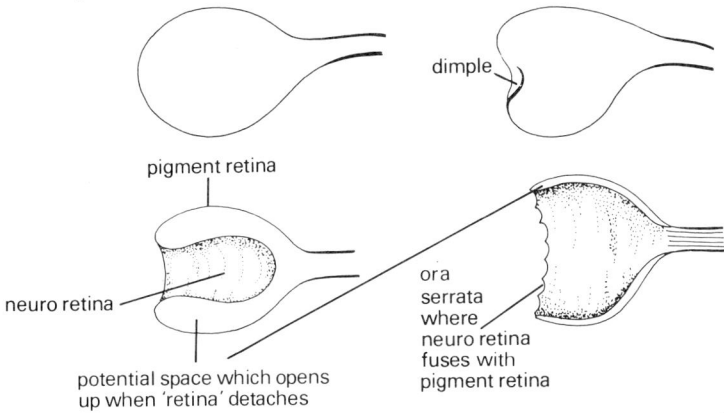

Fig. 15 The development of the neural retina and the pigment retina and the potential space between them

Rods

These spread through the remaining retina. Although clearly working during the waking hours, they come into their own when reduced illumination has deprived the cones of their traditional dominance. This process is known as dark adaptation. It is lost in some retinal diseases, the most famous of which, and happily uncommon, is Retinitis Pigmentosa.

The dark adapted retina, dependent on rods, cannot recognise colour, and it is this feature which produces that subtle yet heightened perception in the moonlight—those honeyed shadows that daylight sharpens with an unpalatable edge.

As part of the brain, the retina must have a copious blood supply. This derives from two sources: the outer half of the retina is fed from the choroid across the retinal pigment layer; the inner half is fed from the central retinal artery that enters the eye through the optic nerve head. It will come as no surprise that the macular area, being the most highly sensitive, is the one that suffers most when the blood supply is compromised. A retinal detachment, no matter how brief, usually blunts the edge of macular vision. The uncertain blood supply of later years becomes more obvious at the macula than in the remaining retina.

FOCUSING MECHANISMS

So far we have dealt with light entering the eye, but no mention yet has been made of how this light is directed to the relevant parts of the retina from various distances. The optical diagrams necessary to demonstrate this—recalled only as unpleasant memories from early days in the physics classroom—have sadly persuaded many people that ophthalmology is but natural philosophy clouded over by medical jargon. The terms long and short sight have done nothing to dispel this cloud. Medicine abounds with confident mis-statements, but none so confidently mis-stated as these.

Anyone who has set fire to dry grass with sunlight through a convex lens will be familiar with the principle of bringing light to a focus from infinity. The convention is that such light is drawn with parallel rays. The nearness of the focal point to the surface of the lens depends essentially on its strength.

Normal sight
This eye will bring parallel rays of light to a focus on the macula without any effort by its focusing muscles (Fig. 16). For ophthalmic

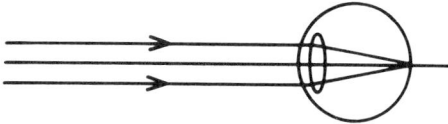

Fig. 16 The normal sighted eye (emmetropic)
       Sees in the distance without effort

purposes anything further off than 6 m is infinity. This explains why normal distance visual acuity is recorded as 6/6 (20/20 ft). The upper figure is the distance at which the test card is being looked at. The lower figure is the distance at which that letter size ought to be seen. 6/12 means that at 6 m distance the eye in question could only record a letter size which should have been seen at 12 m (Fig. 17).

Near vision
Similar to a camera, an eye can pull its focus from infinity to less than 6 m. It achieves this by contraction of the ciliary muscle. This allows the naturally elastic lens capsule to increase the thickness of the lens and hence to shorten its focal length. The actual distance chosen to read varies with habit, and indeed the length of the arm, and is not included in the assessment of near vision. Any test merely records the ability of the eye to discern print of diminishing size (Fig. 18).

As the years go by the lens hardens and fails to respond to directions

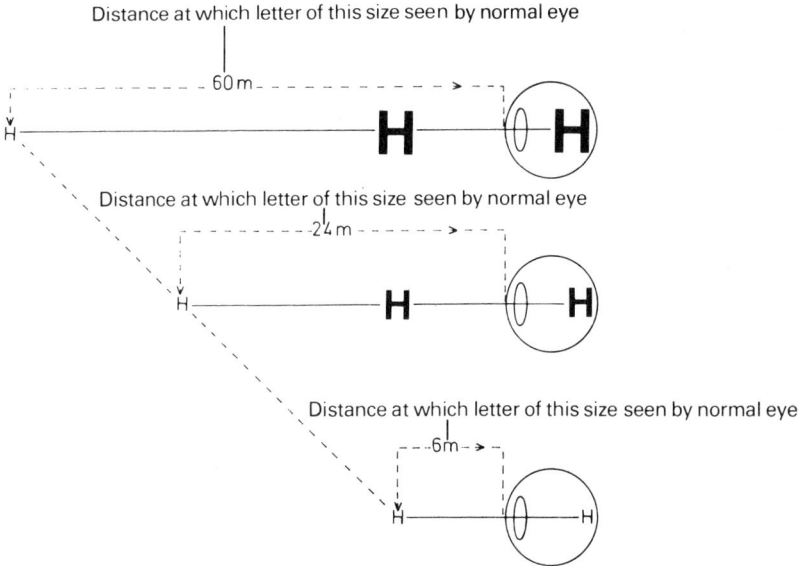

Distance at which letter of this size seen by normal eye

60 m

Distance at which letter of this size seen by normal eye

24 m

Distance at which letter of this size seen by normal eye

6 m

Fig. 17 What the fractions recorded from the Snellen chart mean

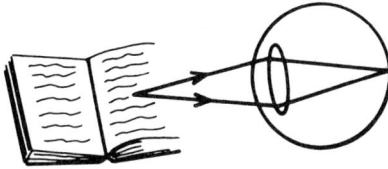

Fig. 18 The normal sighted eye
    Focuses for near by making its lens more convex. The pupil constricts
incidentally at the same time

from the ciliary muscle. Beginning in the early twenties, this process becomes recognisable only in the mid-forties, when people resist the discovery that their arms are becoming too short for visual comfort. *Presbyopia* is the name given to this unfortunate discovery. It increases with age, when lenses of increasing strength are required to compensate for the focusing power lost by the lens of the eye itself (Fig. 19).

Long sight
When the average member of the public talks of long sight, it is normal sight that he really means. The term long sight is taken to imply miracles of distance vision. In fact a sufficiently marked degree of long sight can prevent any effective vision at all.

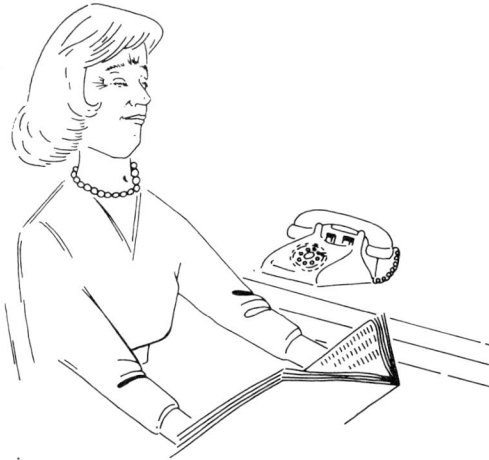

Fig. 19 Presbyopia
The denied evidence of advancing years

The long sighted eye (Fig. 20) has a focal length that is too long for the available eye. Left to its own devices the focal point would lie behind the retina. In order to bring distant rays of light to focus on the retina, the eye has to start working its ciliary muscle. The long sighted eye therefore may see in the distance, but it has to start using up its reading focus to achieve this.

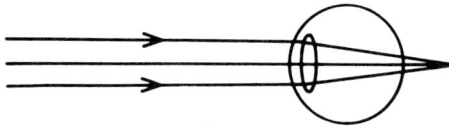

Fig. 20 The long sighted eye (hypermetropic)
Has to make its lens more convex to see in the distance. There may be no range of focus left when it tries to see for near

It is not surprising, therefore, that when it comes to read, it may have used it all up. Thus a thirty-year-old with long sight may find reading impossible and require a lens to correct the distance vision, which will then allow the normal range of focus of the eye to bring reading print into view at the common reading distance.

Short sight

Short sight means many things to many people, and most of them too are wrong.

The focus of this eye is too short for the eyeball (Fig. 21). Parallel rays of light from the distance come to a focus between the lens and the retina, sometimes giving a blurred hint of things of interest,

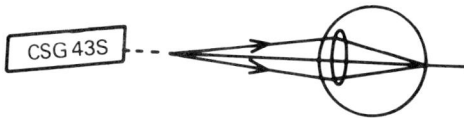

Fig. 21 The short sighted eye (myopic)
      Cannot see in the distance at all. The relaxed focus may be already close enough
to the eye for effortless reading

sometimes not even that. The object in view, therefore, has to be brought closer to the eyeball so that the rays of light diverging from it will push the focal point near enough the retina to be of use. Such eyes see near objects without effort, but pay the price of seeing little in the distance no matter what the effort. It is thought that such a defect may have an influence on short sighted people, making them bookish, withdrawn and unaggressive. It is hard to strike a martial posture when injury to the spectacles may in a flash obscure the supreme moment of glory.

However some doughty warriors have resolved this dilemma by marching to war without glasses at all. Indeed during the Crimean campaign one such pointed a heroic sword at the Heights of the Alma, then led his brigade through an adjacent column from his own army. The Russians, staring in astonishment at this advancing rabble, lost their nerve before what they felt must be a new and irresistible tactical formation.

Astigmatism
All the foregoing refractive errors, as they are called, assume that the eye is a perfect sphere. Occasionally it is not, and sometimes the actual lens within the eye itself does not act equally in all meridians. It might be helpful to imagine such an eye as shaped like a rugby ball. It can never produce a point of focus, either on the retina or off it. If one meridian be sharp, the other by definition must be blunted, also in the manner of an oval. A cylindrical lens that corrects in one meridian only is necessary to correct this error, which will be long or short depending on the total size of the eyeball.

SUMMARY

The normal sighted eye can bring parallel rays of light to focus on the retina without effort.

      Diverging rays of light nearer than 6 m can be brought to focus with an effort that increases with the amount of their divergence. After the mid-forties the hardened lens fails to respond to the ciliary muscles, and reading glasses are thus necessary.

The focal length of the long sighted eye is too long for the eyeball, such an eye having to work, as for reading, in order to see in the distance.

The focal length of the short sighted eye is too short for the eyeball. Such an eye, therefore, can never see in the distance at any time, with or without effort.

The astigmatic eye can never be in focus at any time because it is effectively oval.

The only way in which an eye can overcome these errors without glasses is to call upon the eyelids. If these are contracted sufficiently to form a slit then all the peripheral rays of light will be eliminated, allowing through only the axial rays. These axial rays are undeviated. Although saving may be made at the optician, a price is paid for this vision that outweighs the cost of a pair of spectacles. It means that no-one ever checks for the presence of treatable disease, mainly glaucoma. The physical effort of the eyelids leads to headache and reduced illumination and etches in the skin around the eyes—crow's feet which may add interest to the face but raise speculation about the date of birth despite disguisng cosmetics.

Yet correcting lenses have never been short of opponents. Even today there are those who fiercely condemn them as an outrage against the body. They foretell an ethereal new vision to be revealed to myopes, presbyopes, hypermetropes and astigmatics who have the courage to abandon their glasses and return to nature. Any inconvenient hint that the outlines of nature are now perhaps not quite as sharp as they used to be, is airily dismissed on the grounds that as a heresy it now cannot possibly be true. If there be any heresy it is the persuasion of the credulous that an act of will can transform a faculty they have been born with into one that they would like. There is no virtue in seeing badly if glasses make it possible to see well. Poor vision has nothing to recommend it at any time, and even less when inflicted needlessly on the gullible with counterfeit promises of visual paradise.

3

What patients complain of

A limited number of symptoms are available for distribution through a limitless number of eye problems. The more talkative patients can use them all up, and embellish them as well, even when there is nothing wrong. The confident adherence to one symptom should be taken at its face value, whilst a diffuse attachment to all of them might tell more about the personality than about the eye. When it comes to personal ailments, normally brief and articulate adults disappear behind a smoke screen of their own making—a blend of malapropisms, fabrication and sheer terror.

It is perhaps because statements do not always mean what they say that doctors will never be wholly displaced by diagnostic machines, which respond only to black and white and fail to pick up the shadings so obvious to a sensitive observer.

Ophthalmic symptoms cluster around five main branches:

1. *Alteration in appearance*
2. *Pain*
3. *Disturbance of the lacrimal apparatus*
4. *Visual disturbance*
5. *Double vision*

Only two of these are strictly ophthalmic—visual disturbance and double vision. Normal appearances are well known throughout the body, and any variation should be evident. Pain can occur anywhere. The lacrimal apparatus is really a lubricating gland and drainage system that happen to lie beside the eye.

ALTERATION IN APPEARANCE

Conditions of sudden onset, like a red eye, are obvious. Most people, however, fail to recognise gradual changes in their looks. It is usually left to helpful friends to point out such blemishes. There are several departures from the standard which are accepted as normal. An inventory of theses could be readily constructed, but would be as readily forgotten. Observation is the thing, and as Sherlock Holmes stated: 'Looking does not necessarily mean seeing'.

PAIN

Aches in the eye, stabbing pains through the eye, a sensation of pressure behind the eye—such frequent symptoms share the common feature that the cause almost always lies somewhere else—not least in the paranasal sinuses. To complete this trail of false impressions, acute glaucoma, the most serious ocular emergency of them all, is as likely to cause pain in the forehead or indeed in the belly, as in the eye. *The unrelenting rule is to look at the eye in the same way every time; the presence of signs means that the cause is in the eye; the absence of signs means that it is not.*

If pain follows use of the eyes, then it is fair to ascribe this to some uncorrected refractive error. Morning headaches are not caused by refractive errors, unless insomnia has lead to reading in the night.

DISTURBANCE OF THE LACRIMAL APPARATUS

People may complain of dry eyes when the lacrimal gland has ceased to produce in later life what it used to produce in early life. The rheumatic disorders are notorious for bringing this about at an earlier age.

Watering follows blockage of the drainage apparatus, which may occur anywhere from ill-fitting eyelids down to the nasolacrimal duct. Watering may also follow some sort of irritation to the eyes or the eyelids, and should this be infiltrated with purulent discharge then clearly we have moved into the realms of infection.

VISUAL DISTURBANCE

Since the eye is an extension of the brain, it is reasonable to describe disturbances of vision just as we might describe disturbances of the central nervous system.

Firstly, normal function may be distorted in some way.

Secondly, there may be extra features in the vision which should not be there.

Thirdly, there may be loss of features from the vision which should be there.

Visual distortion
Complaints of this usually mean that the central vision is not quite up to standard. Common causes are macular degeneration or cataract.

Photophobia

Dislike of light affects inflamed eyes, or those with insufficient pigment to absorb excess illumination—albinism. Patients with viral infections and migraine share this dislike, and neurotics are frequently to be found advertising their desire for anonymity behind opaque sunglasses.

Features which ought not to be present

Haloes

Should the cornea become oedematous for some reason, then the patient will be aware of a rainbow ring around lights. Classically this is a warning of an imminent attack of acute glaucoma. Monochromatic haloes, more common than rainbow haloes, mean early cataract. The patient will not make the distinction unless we ask him and if we do not ask, we will not make the distinction either.

Flashing lights

The visual pathway from the retina to the occipital cortex is a system designed to respond with a sensation of light to visual impulses. Because of its high degree of specialisation it responds with the same sensation to other impulses as well. These may range from breaks in the retina to tumours in the temporal lobe.

Floaters

Normal degeneration of the vitreous gel, happening in the fullness of time, leaves little strands and wisps in the vitreal cavity that become visible and often a trial to their possessor. Sudden and recent onset obviously implies some active process. In a transparent organ, this may be due to inflammatory cells or fragments of traumatic debris.

Features which ought be present but are not

Transient loss of vision

Some defects in the cerebral blood flow, or in the ocular blood flow, will produce an instant dimming of the corresponding visual field. This symptom must always be taken seriously.

Field defects

Any lesion known to general pathology may impinge upon the visual pathway. They do not, however, impinge upon consciousness unless they are of sudden onset. Most common is chronic glaucoma, quietly eroding the visual field while people bask in the false security of normal central vision.

DOUBLE VISION

Allegations of double vision frequently turn out to be simple blurring, and as such belong to the previous section.

However, genuine double vision can mean one of two things. If it occurs with only one eye open, then something—usually cataract—has split the light entering the eye (monocular diplopia).

If it happens with both eyes open, then some opacity may still have split the light in one eye, but more likely the eyes will have suddenly begun to point in different directions. This must mean a paralysed muscle until full ocular movements prove otherwise. Children squinting, or adults who started life as children with the same sort of squint, cannot suffer double vision because their eyes do not work together.

SUMMARY

Cosmetic changes are usually self-evident.

Authentic ocular pain will have an obvious ocular basis.

Deficient tears lead to a dry irritable eye that may become infected and paradoxically may begin to water.

Simple watering follows deficient drainage.

Ocular symptoms, like symptoms anywhere else, can be directed by simple questioning into recognisable categories. It is occasionally helpful, but not as helpful as all that, to ask what opinion patients had of their vision before seeking advice. It is surprising how little people actually know of their own eyes. Even their alleged vision from Army days can be deceptive, for in times of national emergency there was an excusable tendency for military doctors to hurry monocular conscripts into uniform. To be fair, some eager combatants compounded the deception by memorising the test chart while the doctor was at his paper work.

Double vision usually turns out not to be double vision at all: the term is commonly misused to describe blurred vision. Monocular double vision is due to some opacity in the transparent media. Binocular double vision means that some factor either transient or permanent has mechanically taken the eyes outside the range over which the extra-ocular muscles normally hold them together.

4

How to elicit essential signs

When people embark on some extended project, their confidence with the bits they know is eaten away by their constant pre-occupation with the bits they do not know or feel they do not know. While only half their mind is available at any one moment for productive use, the other half is distracted with unproductive doubts.

This might be a fair description of ophthalmic examination. We know all about reading charts, but when our patient fails to see any letters, we are not quite sure what to do next.

We know an ophthalmoscope is required to see the back of an eye, but falter when it does not produce the expected picture. However, we tend not to know that a simple torch and a good history can give a safe diagnosis in most cases.

In the interests of perfection there has been a perfectly understandable tendency to all specialities to include all possible symptoms and signs on the way to diagnosis. This is praiseworthy. However, its worth may not be instantly evident to those who are instructed in another specialty, or in that complex of specialties which we call general practice.

In our concern to give equal weight to every little feature, we may miss or forget or misinterpret the big ones. The difference between moderate watering and slight watering is not always obvious—after all how long is a piece of string?

This vogue for completeness reached its apogee with a large square slide rule issued by a drug firm some years ago. All conceivable causes of the red eye were paraded along the upper edge of the square. Every square centimetre of the slide was taken up by every imaginable clinical feature. The front was perforated by a series of windows where appeared the diagnosis as the rule slid back and forth in permutation between the clinical features and the disease. Meanwhile along the lower edge appeared the appropriate remedy, quite by chance manufactured by the same company.

The idea was well intentioned but came to grief by its very complexity and by the choice of material, which collapsed with use.

With time it became difficult to decide where the slide actually belonged. One millimetre too little or one millimetre too much and we had an elegantly boxed corticosteroid preparation recommended for a condition where anything but was indicated.

Ophthalmic examination can be reduced to a handful of simple elements. We have agreed that a careful look at a normal face can give a standard base line against which any variation can be measured. Thereafter we require a way of determining whether failure to see will respond to a pair of glasses or not. This is perfectly possible, while understanding nothing whatsoever about lenses. It may be the first step to a diagnosis, for it is mandatory to explain why a patient does not see as well as he ought to, or used to.

We then require a simple test to determine the state of the visual field in each eye.

We require signs to distinguish the serious causes of the red eye from the less serious causes, and from each other, without ambiguity.

The pressure of the eyeball may be estimated roughly without instruments. The ocular movements, if the history suggests it necessary, can be measured, not as an ophthalmic examination but as part of the general cranial nerve examination.

Finally we come to the ophthalmoscope, which allows a view of the posterior pole of the eyeball. In practical terms this means the optic disc, the macula and the vessels adjacent to the optic disc.

Naturally other methods exist to take the diagnosis to a specialist level, but that is what specialists are for.

CENTRAL VISION

This splits naturally into two groups—distance and near.

The Snellen Chart (distance vision)

This chart operates on the principle that the nearer something is to the eye the bigger it appears, and vice versa. An object seen at 6 m will subtend a rather larger angle in the eye than the same object seen at 12 m.

The Snellen Chart offers a series of letters of decreasing size, and a patient is asked to say what they are, using only one eye at a time (see Fig. 17).

If the vision be normal, the patient will see at 6 m (20 ft) what ought to be seen at 6 m. Failure to make out the letters at the correct distance does not necessarily imply that the eyes are in poor health. They may need a pair of glasses. Indeed, considering the extensive range we accept as normal, it is surprising that more people do not make use of available corrections.

Corrective lenses, however, are the province of the eye specialist, but it is still easy and possible for anyone to distinguish visual loss due to refractive error from visual loss due to something else. The device used—it is hardly an instrument—is the pinhole disc (Fig. 22A & B).

Fig. 22A The pinhole disc
       An infallible method to tell if poor central vision (for distance and near) is due to a spectacle error or not

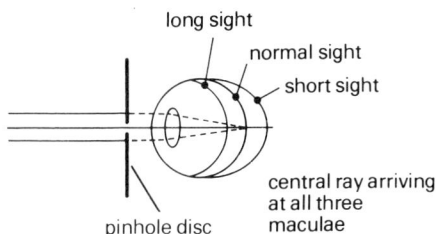

Fig. 22B How the pinhole disc works

The pinhole disc

The principle is absurdly simple. Of the rays of light presented to an eye, all bar the central are deviated out of line by the focusing power of that eye. The central ray however is not deviated because there is nothing to deviate it and so it must reach the macula no matter what the refractive error. In normal circumstances the fact of its passage is overwhelmed by all those other rays that move people to say they cannot see. However the pinhole disc eliminates them all and allows only the central ray to pass on its own. If the macula has the potential to see them the pinhole disc will prove it.

Its use is equally simple. It takes the place of a whole box of lenses and can slip so easily into the pocket that it can slip just as easily out of mind.

Held by the patient about 1 in before the eye under examination, whilst the other is covered, almost magically it will turn a vision of 6/60 into one of 6/6.

There is only one caveat. Any opacity lying on the axial line, be it a corneal scar or a cataract, must be exaggerated by the pinhole disc. This is the only physical obstruction to its use.

The critical value of this little disc cannot be stressed enough.

Near vision

Near vision, which of course demands an element of focus on the part of the eye, can be tested without glasses, but there are one or two circumstances where failure of the eye to read the smallest print does not necessarily mean ill health. It will be remembered that the long sighted eye may have used up all its reading focus in the distance, and that the presbyopic eye has a diminishing, or absent, reading focus related to age. The pinhole disc can be used for near vision as well.

It is important to test near vision, because the eye may still manage the smallest reading print and fail to see the distance chart at all. There may be varying reasons for this, but it will demonstrate a functioning macula.

To avoid confusing the patients, and occasionally ourselves, it is best to use the term *reading* for near, and *seeing* for distance. There is a deplorable tendency to ask people what they can read when presenting them with a distance chart, and it is not surprising to see them pull out their reading spectacles and declare impending blindness.

The E test

It must be remembered that some people cannot read at all, whether owing to extreme youth or to misfortune. It is still possible to test visual acuity by presenting them with a capital letter E. They are then asked to look at a chart covered with this same letter, all pointing in different directions. If they can demonstrate the direction of selected letters then it can be assumed that they are seeing this letter, and the visual acuity registered accordingly.

FIELD OF VISION

Peripheral field loss is usually allowed to run unchecked until the centre is affected. There are machines for plotting accurately the normal visual field, but a pair of hands can form a very simple screening test. It is simple and obligatory to check the hand movement field on everybody who complains about their eyes, even if it is only the central vision they are likely to be complaining about.

The visual pathways

These run anatomically from the retinae along the optic nerves, the optic chiasma, the optic tracts and the optic radiations to the occipital cortex of the brain. Each visual field, which it will be recalled looks like a pear on its side, the short stalk pointing inwards, is split into a temporal half and a nasal half. This split takes place vertically through the fixing point of central vision. The temporal half of each retina is represented in the visual cortex of its own side. The nasal part of each retina crosses over to the opposite side at a junction known as the optic chiasma. It then continues backwards to be represented in that occipital cortex. This chiasma is very closely related to the pituitary gland and the internal carotid artery.

The arrangement is simpler than it looks, and not merely designed by Nature to protect her mysteries. Everything seen by the retina lies in the field opposite to the physical part of the retina involved. Thus objects on the floor will be seen by the upper retina, those to the temporal side by the nasal retina, and so on.

It should be now clear that the nasal half of one eye and the temporal half of the other eye cover the visual field on the opposite side of the body.

In general terms, lesions anterior to the chiasma must affect one eye only. Lesions at the chiasma classically damage the crossing nasal fibres from each eye, giving rise to temporal field defects on each side. Lesions behind the chiasma catch the temporal fibres from one side plus the nasal fibres from the opposite side, and will thus affect the corresponding field of each eye (a homonymous defect)—temporal for one eye, nasal for the other.

The confrontation field

No instrument other than the hands are needed to perform this test (Fig. 23). With one eye closed, or preferably covered, the patient is asked to look directly at the eye of the examining doctor. The doctor then, with an awareness of his own pear-shaped field, flaps both hands at the same time, first in the upper field and secondly in the lower field, in a position corresponding to the extremities of a St Andrew's cross. Clearly the test must be performed with a suitable gap between patient and doctor to allow the hands to be visible. It must also be performed with a certain conviction, for the hands fluttering down from the upper to the lower extremities of the cross are not unlike the manoeuvres of a witch doctor supplicating for rain.

We now turn to the physical eye, pausing only to register the position of the lids, and any apparent variations. There are now two vital observations to be made, and a third subtle one. These observations must be made every time. A relentless repetition over a short space of time will make this examination ritual second nature. There are after all not many elements to remember. One leads on to the next, and indeed after a while all three may be made at once.

1. *The state of the cornea.*
2. *The state of the pupil.*
3. *The depth of the anterior chamber.*

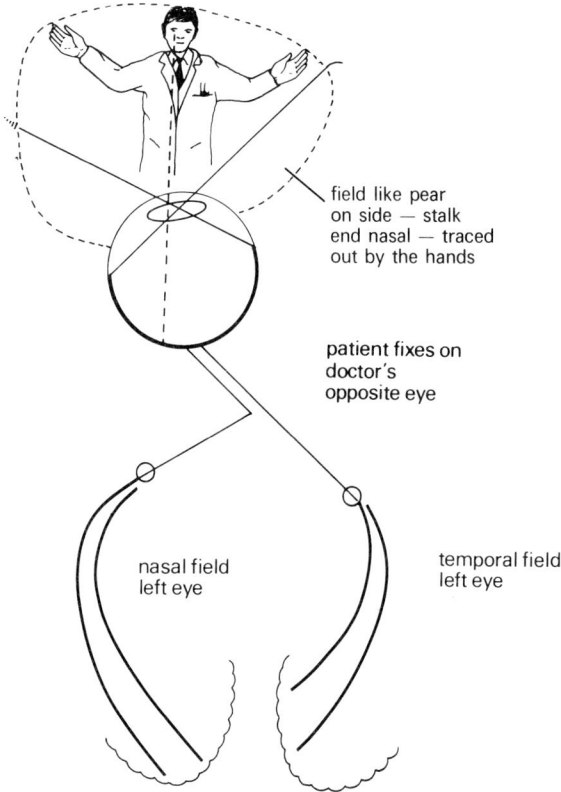

field like pear
on side — stalk
end nasal — traced
out by the hands

patient fixes on
doctor's
opposite eye

nasal field
left eye

temporal field
left eye

Fig. 23 How to test the visual field by confrontation
    As important as the pinhole disc. If the doctor tries to cover one of his own eyes
he will find himself attempting with two hands a manoeuvre for which he clearly needs
three. The ensuing charade may be too much for his patient

CORNEAL LUSTRE

The front surface of the cornea glistens and sparkles in youth,
although turning with ill health and age into the familiar lack-lustre
eyes of the elderly—as though decades of watching human activity
have dulled the eye as well as the spirits. A circle of white (the arcus
senilis) separated by a small distance from the sclera, may encircle the
cornea, giving the impression of reduction of ocular size (see Fig. 36).

Diseases affecting the cornea, classically a corneal abrasion or ulcer, will frequently result in a break of the anterior layer. This may be visible to simple examination with a torch, but without doubt will be visible when the broken areas are outlined accurately with a dye known as sodium fluorescein. A small magnifying lens makes these observations easier, and gives them a certain professional aura.

Sodium fluorescein
Coming as either a liquid or as an impregnated strip of paper, this is another easily carried piece of equipment and a highly vital one. The liquid is perhaps less happy in use than the strip, because as well as staining the eye it will stain everything else it comes in contact with. The paper in theory should be moistened with some sterile isotonic solution, but water from a tap is reasonably adequate. A red eye is usually so moist anyway that extraneous moistening may be superfluous. The tip can then be stroked along the inner surface of the lower lid, allowing the dye to fill the conjunctival sac.

A green colouration will now wash across the cornea, picking up in special detail any areas where the corneal epithelium is broken.

THE PUPIL REFLEXES

The pupil is that hole in the centre of the iris which changes in size in response to various stimuli. It has two muscles. The more powerful, a sphincter running around its margin, makes the pupil smaller when it contracts and larger when it relaxes. Active constriction is mediated via the parasympathetic nervous system.

The weaker muscle—the dilator pupillae—runs from this round muscle outwards to the periphery of the iris. Active dilatation, mediated via the sympathetic nervous system, reinforces the dilatation started by the relaxing sphincter. The pupil regulates the amount of light entering the eye, constricting in the sunlight, dilating at dusk, and decreasing in size when active near vision is called for to allow a greater precision of focus.

There are thus two distinct reflex pathways—one in response to light, the other in response to near focus (accommodation). The former is by far the more important.

The light reflex
As with other reflexes there is a neuromuscular response to a stimulus. There is an inflow pathway and an outflow pathway.

The stimulus is light which, falling on the retina, travels by the optic nerve along the optic tract to the lateral geniculate body at the level of the mid brain. Because the inflow does not rise above this level the pupil reflexes can remain intact, although destruction of the occipital cortex has made the patient blind.

Connection is made in the mid brain, from which the outflow pathways proceed along each third cranial nerve to the sphincter muscle of each iris. It is for this reason that illumination of one eye makes both pupils constrict. The constriction on the same side is known as the direct light reflex. That of the fellow eye is known as the consensual light reflex (Fig. 24).

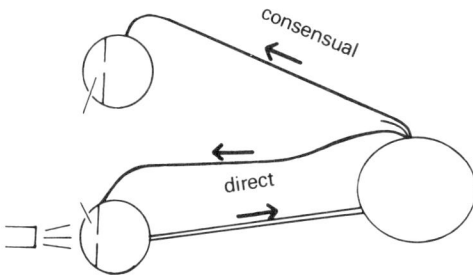

Right eye exposed to light: both pupils constrict

Fig. 24 The pupil light reaction
Both respond when one is exposed to a bright light

The accommodation reflex

Although clearly this must have an inflow pathway, it is as yet unknown despite much imaginative speculation. It has been suggested that contraction of the medial rectus muscles converge when the eyes read sparks off the inflowing impulse. The outflow can be considered the same as that of the light reflex.

Inflow defect

Disturbance at any point along the inflow pathway eliminates or reduces the inflow stimulus on that side. The result is poor constriction of the pupil on the affected side—the direct reflex—and on the opposite—the consensual reflex.

Similar testing of the normal fellow eye will produce normal direct and consensual reflexes.

Outflow defect

Disturbance at any point along the outflow pathway will result in reduced constriction on the affected side, no matter which eye is illuminated.

DEPTH OF THE ANTERIOR CHAMBER

The eclipse test

A vital sign to elicit, upon it depends our ability to state categorically the imminent danger or freedom from acute glaucoma—one of the three major causes of the red eye.

A light directed from the margin of the cornea across the iris plane will illuminate as much of the anterior chamber as its depth allows. In a deep anterior chamber the entire iris will be suffused with light. In a shallow anterior chamber (Fig. 25)—the kind that may give rise to acute glaucoma—only the half adjacent to the light will be illuminated. The remote half is in shadow—the light is eclipsed.

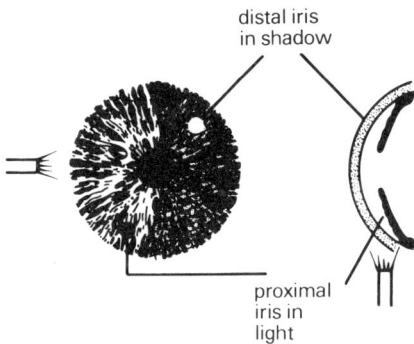

distal iris
in shadow

proximal
iris in
light

Fig. 25 The Eclipse test
Failure to observe whether or not the anterior chamber is shallow is negligence

INTRA-OCULAR PRESSURE

Thoughts of acute glaucoma should put one in mind of a tense eyeball with more aqueous than it can cope with, and hard to touch. Before we can say that the pressure is raised, we must have a method of arriving at this conclusion.

Tonometry is the name given to this manoeuvre, whether it be done by fingers or by instruments. The latter are best left to the ophthalmologist.

Digital tonometry

The basic principle is to palpate the eyeball for fluctuation, like a boil. It is, however, important to palpate the eye and not the tarsal plate, which will lead to a diagnosis of glaucoma every time. Palpation therefore must be done above the tarsal plate with the eye looking downwards.

The easiest way is to lean on the patient's forehead with the ring fingers, brushing the middle or index fingers while palpating the 'boil', as in Figure 26. In the good old days before instruments were available, the shortcomings of this test were given a spurious elegance by the Latin title *tactus eruditis*. Spurious though it may be, it is more elegant than tonometry done badly with an instrument, and fingers are not in need of regular calibration. Indeed it takes regular use to become familiar with the instruments. A false reading is still a false reading, and not more scientific than a finger tension, even though it be recorded in millimetres of mercury.

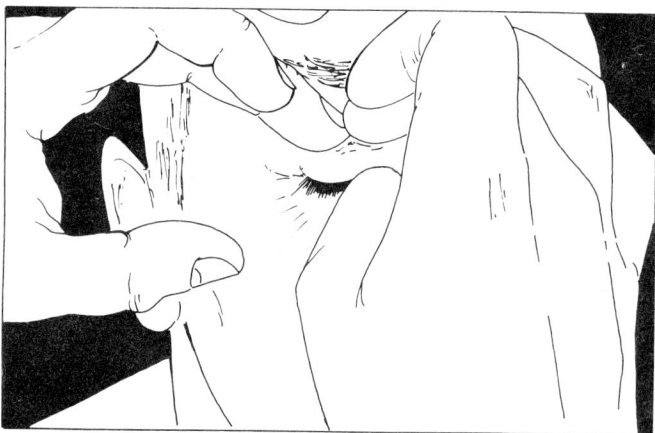

Ring fingers leaning on forehead pressure taken by middle fingers palpating globe like a boil above outer margin of tarsal plate

Fig. 26 Finger tension
The ring or middle fingers are brushed together alternately pulp to nail

LOOKING AT THE FUNDUS

We come at last to the direct ophthalmoscope. Ophthalmoscopy started in the middle of the 19th century when Helmholtz rediscovered what the medical press of 30 years previously had ignored when described by Purkinje—a man whose entire life seems to have been spent making medical discoveries that have brought other people fame.

In principle, light is introduced through the pupil to illuminate the back of the eye. The illuminated fundus is then viewed through a small aperture. Were everyone normal sighted that would be the end of it, but errors of refraction in both doctor and patient have to be corrected.

Each ophthalmoscope, if worthy of its name—and there are many—must contain a disc of lenses which can be rotated one way or the other to compensate for myopia or hypermetropia. Clockwise rotation brings the focus up to the instrument. Anti-clockwise rotation pushes the focus backwards on to the distant retina.

Should the person using the ophthalmoscope also wear glasses, he may choose to leave them on his face or rotate their strength into the ophthalmoscope after discarding them.

The direct ophthalmoscope can be a versatile instrument serving not only as a useful light source, but as a means of detecting opacities in the cornea, the lens and the vitreous. It is by far the best way to demonstrate cataract. With the instrument set at 2 notches clockwise, the light is directed at the patient's eye at a distance of 8 in. The pupil, especially if dilated, will fill with the red reflex. Any opacities in the cornea, the lens or the vitreous will show up against the red glow, and their position can be determined with equal simplicity (Fig. 27).

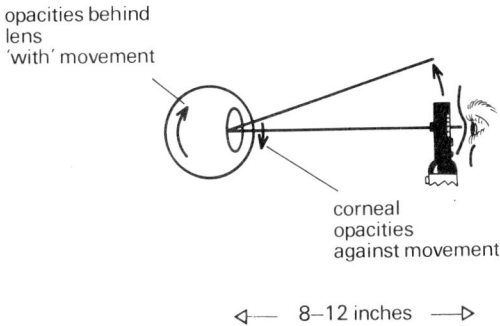

Fig. 27 How to detect opacities through the dilated pupil against the red reflex

When the ophthalmoscope and doctor move slightly from side to side, any opacities will move by parallax. Opacities in the cornea will move against the light; opacities in the lens will not move at all; opacities in the vitreous will move with the light.

The fundus

The optic fundus baffles many people because they are uncertain how to look at it, and equally uncertain what to look at. They almost expect the diagnosis to appear just because they have managed to get the retina into focus and in myopes and aphakics it is not always easy even to do that.

The optic disc should always be looked at en passant whenever anybody complains of eye trouble. This might reasonably be done despite the presence of a lively pupil constricting briskly when the beam is switched on.

As the optic nerves enter the eye at an angle from the nasal side, we will have a better chance of picking them up by directing the beam 'towards the pituitary gland'. The tempting straight on position floods the macula with light, constricts the pupil and leaves us wondering how anyone can ever see anything in the back of the eye, and how we might hide our discomfiture from the patient.

Patients do not help either, because they feel that following the light and the examiner wherever he moves somehow assists in the examination. Opacities in the cornea, the lens and the vitreous heighten this feeling of despair, and increasing age makes the pupil smaller still before the examination is even attempted.

When to dilate the pupil

The rule is perfectly simple. Should the history suggest that a fundal view be obligatory, then the pupil must be dilated with some short acting drug that paralyses the parasympathetic nervous system. Tropicamide 1 per cent will do this and will wear off by the afternoon. Cyclopentolate lasts somewhat longer. An old bottle of Homatropine lurks in most ward cupboards. It should be thrown away before it has the chance to paralyse the patient's focus for some days—an intolerable burden, especially if dilatation of the pupil has failed to produce the expected diagnosis to boot.

As well as Homatropine in the cupboard there lurks in everyone's subconscious the belief that dilating drops should never be used in glaucoma. This translates into practice that they should never be used at all—an embargo strengthened by data sheets which so often include glaucoma in their contra-indications.

The embargo applies only to the eyes with a tendency to acute glaucoma—eyes with a shallow anterior chamber, where dilatation of the pupil may suddenly block the drainage angle. Should the eclipse test indicate a deep anterior chamber, as it usually will, then dilatation of the pupil will be safe, and need not be counteracted afterwards.

When the pupil is dilated the next temptation to be resisted is to examine the entire fundus at once. The direct ophthalmoscope, even in the most practised hands, can rarely see much beyond the equator of the eye. In fact the equator may be defined as the limits of view of the direct ophthalmoscope through the dilated pupil. It is therefore at its best around the posterior pole, where three main features come into view:

1. *The optic disc* (the papilla or optic nerve head).
2. *The macula.*
3. *The retinal vessels.*

The normal fundal appearance is that of choroidal blood vessels glowing red. The range of redness however varies with the concentration of these vessels and the weight of the retinal pigment epithelium masking them. Irregular pigmentation mottles the glow. Heavy racial pigmentation almost turns it to a mallard duck green, whilst Albinoid 'pigmentation' allows the pallor of the white sclera to dominate the background.

The abnormal appearances depend very much on what happens to the pigment layer. Atrophy exposes the white sclera—perhaps overlaid by choroidal remnants or perhaps not. Healed inflammation will ring the gap with a rampart of pigment. Active inflammation with its fluffy clouds will obscure not only the sclera but the choroidal glow as well and indeed may spread to obscure the adjacent vitreous gel.

Each feature should be looked at in turn, and as novices we should not be dismayed if looking at them does not tell us very much to begin with.

The optic disc

The normal optic disc, although in fact measuring some 1.5 mm across, appears rather larger when looked at with an ophthalmoscope. It will appear rather larger still in short sighted (myopic) eyes, becoming smaller as the eyes become long sighted (hypermetropic). It presents three main features which devotees of cricket might remember with the letters MCC. For those who regard cricket as the Englishman's substitute for philosophy, the very absurdity of the idea might make the letters memorable (Fig. 28).

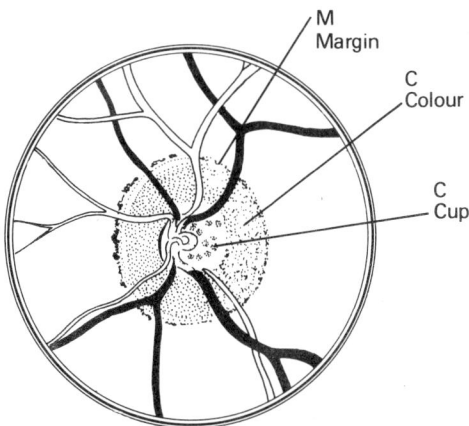

Fig. 28 The normal disc
The adjacent fundal appearance is a truce between the scleral white, reddened and mottled by the choroid, muted by the pigment retina and visible through the neural retina—transparent when it is flat (see Fig. 74)

M—The margin should be sharp in normal eyes, but in small crowded eyes might well be blurred.

C—The colour again will vary according to the size of the eye, being pale in the large myopic eye where the capillaries are less crowded, and darker red in the long sighted eye for the opposite reason.

C—The cup, or cavity, in the centre of the disc takes up about a quarter of its size.

The macula

The absolute centre of this highly sensitive retina—the fovea—lies some 1.5 disc diameters on the temporal side of the temporal margin of the optic disc. It lies in a pit where the retinal layers shelve to allow the maximal amount of light to fall upon the foveal cones and is seen as a glistening dot in the young eye. The paramacular retina is thus heaped up and somewhat thicker than the peripheral retina. This thickening appears still as red, but rather darker than its surroundings.

The retinal vessels

The central retinal artery emerges from the optic disc to spread as arterioles branching and tapering over the entire fundus. Its capillaries feed the half of the retina adjacent to the vitreous, and blood is returned by the retinal venules which follow the arterioles back into the optic disc. The central retinal artery is an end vessel anastamosing with no other arterial system.

The arterioles and venules can be seen forming an arcade around the macula. It is therefore to these three features—the optic disc, the macula and the retinal vessels—that the observer should be directed, while at the same time taking a general view of the red reflex.

SUMMARY

A safe eye is one that will not start to go blind without attracting attention before it is too late. There are but six essential steps to eliminate nagging after-thoughts from the diagnosis of such an eye.

1. Central vision should be assessed for distance and near, if necessary with a pinhole disc. The ability to read the smallest print confirms a functioning macula even though the performance with the distance chart is not impressive.

2. Field of vision can be gauged by confrontation.

3. The corneal surface should glisten and sparkle, and may be

stained by sodium fluorescein to demonstrate any breaks in the epithelium.

4. The pupil reaction to light should follow from the light used to examine the cornea.

5. The depth of the anterior chamber should follow from that again (eclipse test).

6. Finger tension (digital tonometry) should be brought to mind by the association between the eclipse test and acute glaucoma.

The ocular movements need not be looked at unless the history suggests some defect in the ocular muscles.

Only at this point should one think of looking at the back of the eye with the ophthalmoscope, and even that should be delayed until any opacities in the cornea, lens or vitreous have been established. The whole point of ophthalmic examination is to square complaints with findings, and to explain why a patient does not see as well as he should.

The eye like any other tissue suffers when something treatable is missed. Fortunately, however, most disorders will draw attention to themselves because they affect central vision. There are, however, three sinister conditions where a patient can be reassured at one consultation, only to return blind a year later. The first is chronic glaucoma. The second, more rare, is a space-occupying lesion in the pituitary fossa. Both nibble away insidiously at that portion of the vision that people are least conscious of—the visual field. The third is the eye with the shallow anterior chamber—symptomless for the moment, but a potential victim of acute closed angle glaucoma, and liable to explode at any time without warning, often rather less than a year later.

The above system is a simple repetitive ritual that will uncover positive signs where there are those to be uncovered, and although it may not always tell what the condition is exactly, it will always tell what it is not.

There should be no doubt now about when it is safe to dilate the pupil. No ophthalmologist would dream of attempting a diagnosis with the pupil in the way, nor would he begin such an attempt in a sunlit ward with a waning ophthalmoscope.

5

Basic medical principles at work in a special organ

The greatest obstacle to medical learning is the firm belief held by every speciality that it is unique, with a special language and a special importance that places it apart from the common run of all other specialities. In the welter of specifics, sovereign remedies, ancient traditions and eponyms, the common thread that binds them all together is lost. In fact there are more similarities than otherwise. A simple physiology goes wrong, patients complain, doctors interfere, and the only difference is where it all happens.

There is a limited range of things that can actually go wrong. It is the local variation that makes them seem inexhaustible. All tissues can suffer congenital defects, tumours, inflammation, vascular disturbances, and so on. Regional differences add a touch of local colour, but do not change the basic processes.

As an example, inflammation, whatever its cause and whatever its site, will give rise to redness, swelling, pain, heat and loss of function. It may then disappear without trace; it may leave marks of damage in its wake, or it may grumble on as a chronic destructive process. If it happens in the iris then of course it is an ophthalmic problem, but it is inflammation none the less, with all its quirks and all its problems of management (Fig. 29).

This chapter aims to demonstrate, using iritis as an example, how symptoms and signs can be worked out on a reasoned basis, and how on the same reasoned basis a system of management can be evolved. This scheme of symptoms and signs of management can be applied not only to ophthalmic conditions, but to every other medical condition as well.

It will be remembered that the iris is a part of that complex known as the uveal tract. Inflammations of the iris follow the same aetiology as inflammations anywhere else. They may be traumatic, infective, allergic, and most often occur without any demonstrable cause whatsoever.

An acute inflammatory attack, wherever its site, can generally do one of four things.

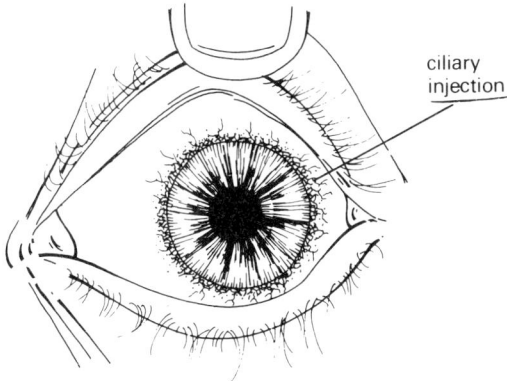

Fig. 29 Iritis
One of the three major red eyes showing inflammation around the corneo-scleral limbus and possibly nothing else

1. *It may resolve without damage to special tissue.*
2. *It may retreat after special tissue has been replaced with functionless fibrous tissue.*
3. *It may spread to an adjacent structure.*
4. *It may continue to smoulder as a chronic disease process.*

The general features of the inside of the eye are known from the first chapter of this book. Combining them with the general principles of inflammation, already common knowledge outside the confines of this book, can produce a practical example of the eye in disease.

1. The blood vessels at the margin of the cornea become inflamed.
2. The iris swells and exudes cells into the anterior chamber.
3. The muscles of the iris sphincter go into spasm, producing a small pupil and some degree of pain.
4. Inflammatory debris dancing about in the visual field can cause tantalising disturbance. It can also deposit silt in the drainage angle, which blocks the flow of aqueous humour.
5. As the inflammation proceeds, adhesions may develop between adjacent structures, most usually the iris and the lens.

None of the preceding information is unpredictable.

DISTURBANCE OF OCULAR PHYSIOLOGY (Fig. 30).

1. The eye drops from its level of perfection as an organ of vision.

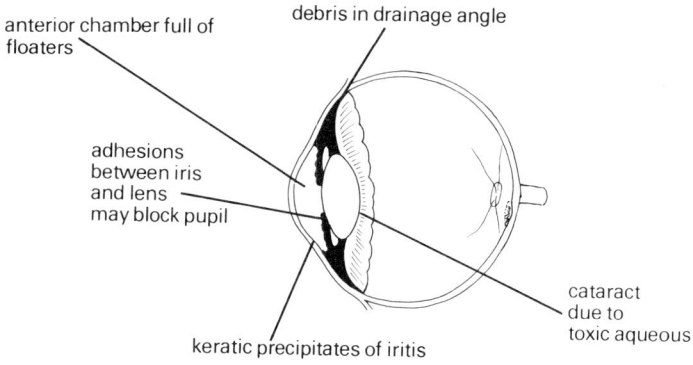

Fig. 30 Iritis
        The possible complications; obstruction of the aqueous flow may not be suspected until the visual field is impaired

2. Adhesions between the iris and the lens may block the flow of aqueous humour.

3. Inflammatory debris in the drainage angle has the same effect. If this blockage be complete, the pressure of the eyeball will rise. If the pressure of the eyeball rises above the blood pressure to the optic nerve head, then it quietly begins to eat away the visual field. We might call this glaucoma, secondary to iritis.

4. If the aqueous humour becomes poisoned by the inflammatory material, it declines in its function as a blood substitute, especially around the lens, which will respond in the only way it can by losing its transparency.

5. Further material deposited on the back of the cornea impairs the function of the endothelial layer, resulting in local oedema of the overlying corneal stroma and epithelium.

If the condition fails to resolve, or does not respond to treatment, then it may destroy the ciliary body, resulting in collapse of the eyeball. It can damage the cornea, resulting in corneal opacification. All these results are predictable.

Clinical findings related to pathology

1. The *central vision* may be affected.
2. The *field of vision* will be normal.
3. The *cornea* should be clear in the early stages. The integrity of its anterior surface can be tested with the dye sodium fluorescein. If the deep surface of the cornea be coated with inflammatory debris (keratic precipitates) then the overlying cornea will appear waterlogged. This will seem to both the patient and doctor to be very

like the translucency of water hosing down a fishmonger's window.

4. The pupil will be small and spastic, unless distorted by the adhesions of a previous attack.

5. The *anterior chamber depth* will not be relevant but its inflammatory aqueous, no longer optically clear, will pick up the beam of a focusing torch in much the same way as dust particles and smoke pick up the projection beam in a cinema. This aqueous flare (Fig. 31) may be the first convincing sign of iritis in an eye with injection around the corneo-scleral limbus and nothing much else to account for it.

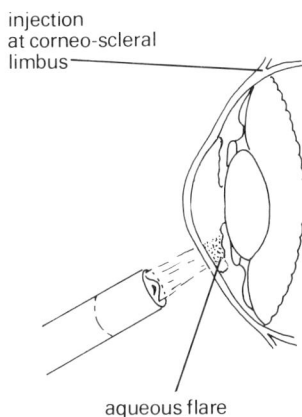

Fig. 31 Iritis
   Aqueous flare. A subtle confirmation of iritis but one easily seen if looked for with a focusing torch: inflammatory debris precipitated from the aqueous may be visible as little white dots on the back of the cornea (Fig. 11)

Management

As with clinical examination, the schemes of management are the same whatever organ is involved. If lack of experience makes us hesitate to do what seems logical, then that is perfectly reasonable. However, it is well to remember that medical advance has not infrequently been the product of persistent logic in the face of orthodox derision. Two examples come to mind.

There was Hickman, the Shropshire veterinarian, who dared suggest that surgery might be more congenial were the patients asleep, especially if they could be wakened up again. His successful demonstration of this on a cow did not bring a trail of admiration to his door. And Semmelweiss, the Viennese obstetrician, lost his reason when his fellow gentlemen accoucheurs refused to believe that the reduced death rate following childbirth in his wards had something to do with antiseptics and water.

Turning from the ironies of history, we can reduce management to a series of principles which are common to all branches of medicine. These may be divided into medical or surgical, short term or long term.

1. *The exciting cause should be removed if possible.*
2. *If the exciting cause is not known then the destructive processes should be curbed if possible.*
3. *The complications should be anticipated. It should be also remembered that remedies frequently have complications also.*
4. *Restoration of function is hopefully the end product of therapeutic intervention.*

It should also be remembered that there is a patient attached to the diseased eye, who is in need of sympathy, comfort, reassurance, and possible analgesics.

The long term aims are much the same as the short term ones, only that the balance inclines towards restoration of function when the drama surrounding the acute illness has subsided.

Although iritis may be associated with conditions like rheumatoid arthritis, or the collagen diseases, the exciting cause is usually not known.

Short term treatment

Provided the cornea is not staining with fluorescein, local drops of corticosteroid may be used to suppress the inflammation and prevent adhesions forming between the iris and the lens. *The frequency of dosage must be tailored to the severity of the condition. Four times daily to the eye has acquired an almost scriptural sanctity, but in many cases every hour would be more appropriate.*

It is not out of place to mention at this point that long term dosage with corticosteroid may be as toxic to the eye as the disease itself. If the iritis poisons the aqueous, so may the corticosteroid, and the lens will respond again by developing a cataract.

Because of the potential adhesions implicit in the inflammatory process, it is to the advantage of the eye to make the development of such adhesions more difficult. If the diameter of the pupil can be increased, this means that the creeping fibrosis has much further to travel. It also means that there is more chance of leaving a gap for the passage of aqueous into the anterior chamber (Fig. 32). The eye also has more chance of seeing through a wide pupil than through a small pupil plastered with inflammatory debris. Therefore the pupil must be dilated with some suitable agent. Atropine drops are time honoured and long acting. They acquire their name of Belladonna

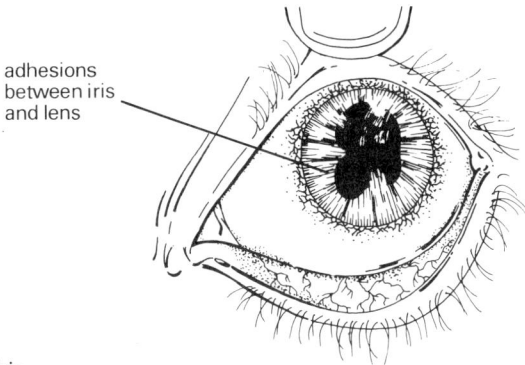

Fig. 32 Iritis
  Adhesions between the iris and the lens. Atropine does not stop this, but it does make the adhesions work harder if they are to block the entire pupil

from the custom of Roman ladies of fashion who added lustre to their eyes by dilating their pupils, for limpid pools, black beneath tremulous lashes, were considered seductive. This was probably true, and for the ladies had the matchless advantage of blurring away the deformities of their more mis-shapen consorts!

  If the flow of aqueous has been disturbed, then the raised intra-ocular pressure has to be brought down. This can be done in two ways. The inflow can be reduced. The outflow can be increased.

  Acetazolamide—a carbonic-anhydrase inhibitor—reduces the production of aqueous. It also affects the production of bicarbonate in the renal tubules, with the resultant danger of a metabolic acidosis—perhaps another reminder of the potential poisons we introduce in the interests of good health.

  Pilocarpine drops for some yet unknown reason increase the outflow of aqueous from the eye. However they also constrict the pupil, which is the one thing we want to avoid in iritis. Their presence, therefore, is not indicated in this condition.

  In the short term we are generally not concerned with perfect function, but we should not forget that the eye will want to see again later. Analgesics may be, and assurance certainly will be, required because all people have an unspoken fear of going blind.

Long term treatment
This applies only to the long term complications of a smouldering chronic iritis. If the pressure of the eye remains high following the disease, this will have to be kept under control with long term anti-glaucoma therapy. If local medications fail then it will be necessary to apply the benefits of surgery.

  This involves cutting a hole in the sclera (Fig. 33) to allow the

aqueous to drain out from the eye. Such a manoeuvre is an outrage to
the body, which naturally tries to close over such an invasion, and
indeed frequently succeeds.

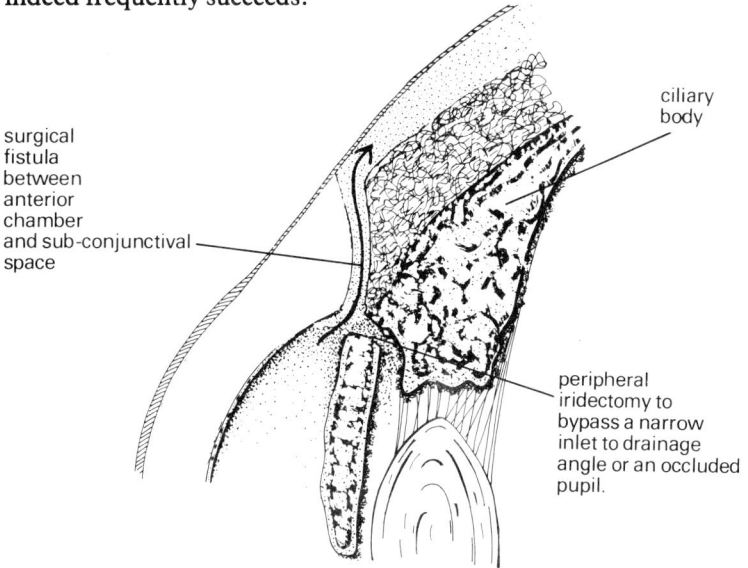

Fig. 33 The essence of a glaucoma operation

If the blockage is at the pupil then a hole may be cut in the iris
(iridectomy) to allow aqueous to drain from the posterior chamber
into the anterior chamber. For some unknown reason the iris never
attempts to heal over these perforations.

Should the lens have succumbed either to the disease or the
treatment, then the eye will not be very useful as an organ of vision.
This might lead us to recommend a cataract extraction, though it
should be remembered that surgery, in the presence of inflammation,
or indeed in the presence of healed inflammation, may induce a fresh
outbreak of the primary disease.

Whatever the basic pathology, the patient will respond with a
limited number of symptoms, and the eye with a limited number of
signs. Awareness of the normal aqueous flow will warn us to beware
for the flow may well cease to be normal with no obvious signs at all.
The ritual of examination will tell us what is wrong or what is not
wrong. The principles of management not unique to the eye will tell
us how to put it right if that be possible. It might also warn us that just
because someone recovers while taking some medication or other,
does not necessarily mean that he recovered because he was taking it.
There is now no reason why we cannot begin to predict what can go
wrong in the eye, and, more to the point, what can be done about it.

6

The external eye

The eyelids, the conjunctiva and the cornea form a natural alliance, working together in health and failing to work together in disease. There is a tendency for the ill effects of this failure to co-operate to spread from the more robust eyelids to the conjunctiva, and finally to the cornea. The cornea tends to keep its personal afflictions to itself, or occasionally may pass them deeper still to involve the iris or even the whole interior of the globe.

The extreme sensitivity of the cornea generally leads all but the most phlegmatic to complain of something. All the available symptoms can appear, but not all at once. Relevant complaints can be easily confirmed by simple observation. But, as ever, their relevance tends to diminish in inverse proportion to the number of things complained of.

Diagnosis is also elementary, provided we can overcome the fear that it should not be so elementary. The secret is to examine all eyes in the same way every time.

Principles of management
The health of the outer eye relies on eyelids snugly fitting, puncta inwards, lashes outwards, and actively blinking—spreading tears from a moist abundant conjunctival sac over a smooth and transparent cornea. Anything that maintains or restores this arrangement without recourse to frank charlatanry can be called treatment.

Medications of one sort or another can be applied to the eye as drops or ointment. Higher concentrations can be achieved by injection underneath the conjunctiva. Systemic dosage may reinforce local treatment. Surgery comes as a last resort, or when the condition is due to some distortion of the normal anatomy.

Drops
Although these have a long and celebrated history, they are not the most efficient way of applying a high concentration of the required drug. As it is unlikely that anything effective remains in the

conjunctival sac for more than a minute after instillation, it will be evident that the sacred dosage of four times a day can have little place in severe conditions of the anterior segment.

Ointments
The major portion is a base of petroleum jelly and liquid paraffin. The more easily soluble the agent, the more effective it will be—and for longer. If overused, they tend to retard the very corneal epithelial regrowth that they seek to promote. However, the disadvantage is misting of vision for a while. People not unreasonably like to see while they are being treated.

Infections
A wide range of organisms can produce infective inflammations. Pyogenic infections most commonly are caused by diplococcus pneumoniae and staphylococcus aureus. Of the viral infections the most important is herpes simplex.

Sulphonamides
Sulphisoxazole 4 per cent and sodium sulphacetamide 10 per cent may still have a place as bacteriostatics against apparent infection. They are effective against some gram positive and gram negative organisms, and are cheap. Problems of resistance do not arise because they are not used systemically. Prolonged usage does not lead to secondary fungal infections.

Antibiotics
A wide range of antibiotics is available for local use, many of which would not be tolerated by the body if given systemically. Chloramphenicol 0.5 per cent is perhaps the most popular and most useful. There is the caveat that the development of allergy would preclude its systemic use were that necessary.

Gentamycin sulphate (0.5–3 per cent) also casts its net on both sides of the gram stain. There are others, but it is better to be sure of two than uncertain about them all.

Clinical perfection demands tests for culture and sensitivity before the start of treatment. Patients with painful eyes may not see it that way, and in practice the report from the laboratory will arrive when the eye is well on its way to recovery. Acute infections should be treated intensively, and the treatment continued for some days after recovery, this being in line with the systemic use of such drugs.

Anti-viral agents
Perhaps the most commonly used is Idox-uridine, available as a drop

for hourly usage and an ointment which may be applied five times daily. There are others available. All these drugs are active against the D.N.A. family of viruses—most especially herpes simplex, although it may also have some activity against herpes zoster. Because of their very action they not only inhibit virus formation, but also the formation of the cells under attack from the same virus. Over short periods thay may destroy viral multiplication, but over long periods may do very much the same thing to the corneal epithelium.

Artificial tears
These are simply long acting moistening agents, which consist essentially of isotonic saline and some viscous material like methylcellulose to prolong their action. The dry eye is vulnerable to infection, and its existence may be overlooked in the general red watering that accompanies such infections. Various proprietary forms share the quality of bland freedom from all noxious chemicals and from allergic reactions.

Corticosteroids
Dexamethazone and Betamethazone figure prominently in ophthalmic preparations. It cannot be said too often that the use of these drugs in the presence of the herpes simplex virus may be the first step to the Law Courts. They have no rival amongst other ophthalmic preparations for their bold contribution to ocular pathology. Yet their frequent prescription is supported by a flawed reasoning that traces back into the mists of our undergraduate subconscious. The sophistical chain might be linked thus:

1. A red eye means inflammation;
2. Inflammation leads to scar formation;
3. Scar formation means an opaque cornea;
4. Corticosteroids suppress inflammation and will prevent scar formation, and hence will maintain corneal clarity;
5. Therefore corticosteroids must be applied to any red eye.

This dangerous fallacy continues to condemn patients to needless and permanent visual loss—hopeful to the end, because they feel better as they continue to get worse.

Corticosteroids must never be instilled into the conjunctival sac until sodium fluorescein has proved the corneal epithelium to be intact.

And as though all this were not enough, corticosteroids have other side effects. Fungal growth also flourishes under the protection of prolonged dosage. The systemic effects of water retention may be paralleled in the eye. Because the eye is not distensible the intra-ocular pressure may rise to dangerous levels. They have also been blamed on less certain grounds for cataract formation.

It might be wondered why, in view of such lethal attributes, there is ever any place for corticosteroids. There are, as in general medicine, certain specific indications, such as iritis, but more often they are turned to in despair when other attempts to whiten an eye have failed. The popular custom of applying a corticosteroid in the shade of an antibiotic has little to recommend it. The former if contra-indicated to begin with, would still be contra-indicated despite the illusory protection of the latter—misguided in prescription, ineffectual in dosage and a potential cause of continued inflammation in its own right.

Oxyphenbutazone

Prepared as an ointment, this substance has the same despairing indication for those grumbling conjunctival inflammations that will not go away with the other remedies. Unfortunately they do not always go away with Oxyphenbutazone either, but the drug does have the advantage of not appearing to favour the growth of the herpes simplex virus.

Astringents

Heavy metal salts of zinc and silver have a long, though not particularly honoured, history in the treatment of persistent oedematous conjunctivitis. Zinc sulphate (0.25 per cent) is available in a variety of proprietary mixtures, and at least makes such eyes more comfortable if not necessarily better. The disadvantage of silver is a deposition of brown staining in the conjunctiva, which disperses slowly and may well cause more anguish than the original condition.

Sodium cromoglycate

This drug, already with some success to its name in the treatment of asthma and hay fever, has a prophylactic rather than a curative action. It is believed to prevent the antigen/antibody combination from disrupting mast cells, thus preventing the release of histamine and similar substances. Although beautifully effective in diagram, with all the potential vasodilators trapped by a defensive ring of chemical formulae, beauty is not always duplicated in life, when some subtle inflammatory combination may escape from this molecular cordon. No serious side effects have been reported to date.

Allergic responses

Unfortunately all drugs, even those used to treat allergy, may give rise to some allergic reactions themselves. Ophthalmic allergies are recognised by the swelling of the tarsal conjunctiva and the skin, and oedema spreading from the lid margins to beyond the orbital limits. As time goes on the skin takes on a leathery sheen, which gives way later to a superficial flaking. No great skill is required to make the diagnosis, and hydrocortisone lotion applied to the skin only, after the offending application has been stopped, will reduce the oedema and ease the patient's resentment.

THE EYELIDS

The eyelids are the mobile part of that protective screen which stretches from the orbital margin to the eyelashes. The outer portion is formed by a delicate elastic skin, which pays the price for its enormous mobility by developing oedema easily in ill health, and maddening wrinkles as the years go by.

Deep to the skin lies a circular striated muscle—the orbicularis oculi—which, on response to impulses from the facial nerve will close the eyelids firmly.

The eye, however, has to open as well, and the upper eyelid is raised by the levator palpebrae superioris, which shares its origin and nerve supply with the superior rectus. A superior tarsal muscle with very much the same action is supplied by the sympathetic nervous system, and by this medium is produced the classic lid retraction when the thyroid overacts.

A fibrous plate deep to the muscle layer gives each lid its firm stability. Deep in these plates are lodged the most important of the lid glands—the meibomian glands which secrete sebaceous lubricants for the inner surface. It is blockage and infection of these glands that produce the classic tarsal cyst. The deep surface of the eyelid is lined by the tarsal conjunctiva. The eyelashes protruding from the outer part of the lid margin have follicles and sebaceous glands at their roots, as do hair anywhere else. Blood flows to the eyelids from the ophthalmic artery. Sensation, as to most other things in that area, is supplied by the first division of the fifth cranial nerve. The lacrimal puncta, at the medial end of the eyelids, drain tears into the lacrimal sac and the nasolacrimal duct.

Malposition of the eyelids

When the eyelids fail to maintain their snug relationship with the globe, then a major link in the arrangement of normality is broken, and the fragile structures dependent on this arrangement begin to suffer.

The lids may separate from the globe (ectropion) due to senility, a facial palsy, contracting scar tissue, or laceration (Fig. 34). The lacrimal punctum floating away with it can no longer pick up tears which begin to flood across the cheek, and in time excoriate the facial skin. The exposed conjunctiva becomes keratinised, and the cornea,

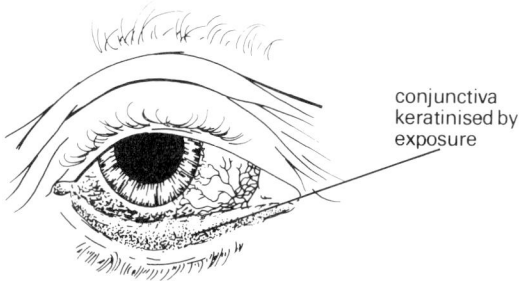

conjunctiva
keratinised by
exposure

Fig. 34 Ectropion
A breach in the alliance of the anterior segment

now also exposed, begins to abandon the delicate privileges of clarity in the interests of sheer survival. Virulent organisms flourishing in the abnormal circumstances may penetrate the globe itself.

When the lids turn inwards (entropion), the abrading lashes add another dimension to the corneal damage.

Management
The fragile tissues must be saved first, infection treated with intensive local antibiotics and corneal exposure soothed with artificial tears. Thereafter the lids must be restored as near as possible to the flawless perfection of youth. Special attention must be given to the lid margin and to the lacrimal canaliculus, where maladroit repair can impose iatrogenic elements on a problem sufficiently difficult to begin with.

Tarsal cyst
A stagnant gland may become infected, ending up as a meibomian abscess. It may then thicken and harden into a small lump (chalazion) which, if large enough, will distort vision (Fig. 35). Infection of course produces its well known signs.

The acute phase requires intensive local antibiotics. The pain may be eased by hot spoon bathing—hot soaked lint wrapped around a wooden spoon applied to the closed eyelids. Although not bacteriologically sound, the same effect may be produced by the lower rim of a hot cup in between mouthfuls of tea.

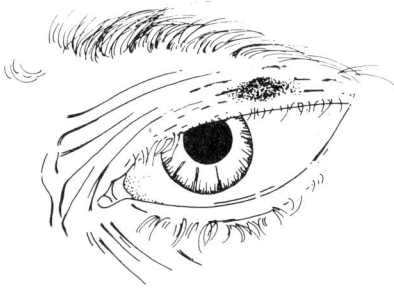

Fig. 35 An infected tarsal cyst
A meibomian abscess frequently mistaken for a stye

Once a cold tarsal cyst has emerged, if large enough, it will require to be removed. This may be done in most cases under local anaesthesia. With the lid held in place by a meibomian clamp, the pointing head can be incised through the tarsal conjunctiva, and the contents rapidly curetted.

Rodent ulcer
Basal cell carcinoma is the most common tumour of the eyelids. A dimpled lump, with rolled edges and indolent or recurring infection that never seems to heal (Fig. 36), it could burrow its way into the skull bones if left to its own devices. Fortunately its peculiarities are well enough known to prevent such negligent delay, when radio-therapy or simple excision should put an end to its significance. The implications of its proximity to the lacrimal punctum should be obvious.

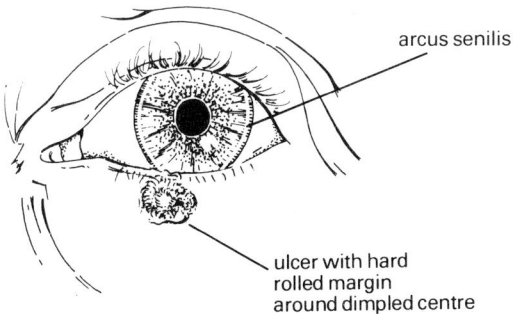

arcus senilis

ulcer with hard
rolled margin
around dimpled centre

Fig. 36 A rodent ulcer (basal cell carcinoma)
The white arcus senilis is an unrelated reminder that the likely victim is beyond middle age

Epicanthus

A vertical fold of skin hiding the medial end of the eyelids can give the false impression of an ingoing squint. Its inconsequence will become more apparent in the relevant chapter.

Ptosis

When the upper lid fails to rise above the pupil line, the explanation must vary with age, the mode of onset and any associated features. Children clearly suffer the congenital variety, although adults may just have to put up with it for a long time. In childhood, ptosis may prevent the development of binocular vision and may also be associated with a vertical squint, threatening binocular vision in its own right. Surgery may therefore be required to allow vision to develop. It may also be required for cosmetic reasons, though the successful exposure of a depressed eye may not always be greeted with enthusiasm by the patient or his parents.

Structures that defy gravity in youth tend to droop with age, and the upper lid is a classic example (Fig. 37). Both congenital and senile ptosis are characterised by the total absence of sinister symptoms and by intact cranial nerves.

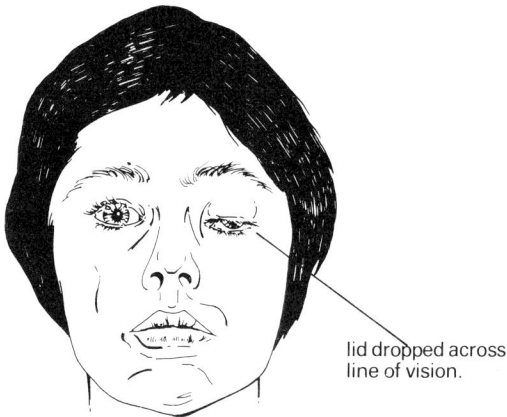

lid dropped across line of vision.

Fig. 37 Ptosis

However the sudden onset of a dropped lid means that something has gone wrong with either the third cranial nerve or the cervical sympathetic chain.

A third nerve palsy makes the eye virtually immobile, makes the pupil large and raises the disturbing possibility of an intra-cranial aneurysm.

Paralysis of the cervical sympathetic, classically caused by a bronchogenic carcinoma at the root of the neck, does not interfere with the eye movements, and it makes the pupil small. It does not prevent the voluntary muscles from raising the eyelids should they be asked to. This collection of signs is known as Horner's syndrome.

A tick in the eyelids

This trivial flickering of the lids, linked with emotional stress or languor, is called myokymia. The patient becomes convinced that other people notice the twitching as much as he does. The treatment is to assure him that they do not.

However they do notice it when clonic twitching of the eyelids spreads to engulf the muscles on one side of the face. This disturbing sequence, more common in middle aged females, is then not just noticed—it is misinterpreted by males of all ages, who take it for a provocative wink when the mortified victim, caught unawares by her eyelids, is only turning her head away to hide them.

If this clonic facial hemispasm does not resolve spontaneously, it can be weakened by the injection of alcohol into the facial nerve. This may be effective; indeed it may be too effective, and bring the patient back with facial muscles that, far from twitching, fail to move at all.

The eyelashes

Infection of one lash root forms the classical stye (Fig. 38). Chronic infection of more than one lash root sheds the scales of blepharitis which must be removed to allow antibiotic penetration to break the cycle of infection.

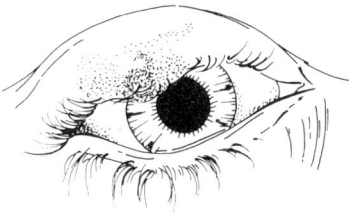

Fig. 38 Stye
Infection of a lash root

Lashes pointing in the wrong direction (trichiasis) can destroy the cornea. Aberrant lashes may reasonably be plucked out with epilation forceps, unfortunately only to return in a more wiry and vigorous growth. Electrolysis down each hair follicle is a despairing alternative to epilation.

Should the number of lashes defeat one's patient, then the entire row may be turned away from the eye by surgery. A line cut behind the row of lashes may be filled in with buccal mucous membrane. The cosmetic short-comings of the procedure and the painful mouth will seem as nothing compared with the intense ocular relief that follows the operation.

THE CONJUNCTIVA

The conjunctiva is that translucent lining which acts as the 'synovial membrane' for that part of the eyeball which has to make its movements exposed to the air.

It lines the deep surface of the eyelids (the tarsal conjunctiva). From there it curves backwards all around the eye for a distance of 2 cm, when it changes direction to come forwards again, this time coating the eyeball (the bulbar conjunctiva). The membrane is loose and thrown into folds, and the major fold where it changes direction to form a blind ended sac is known as the conjunctival fornix. Consisting of two layers, an epithelium of cylindrical cells and a substantia propria of goblet cells, it becomes continuous with the corneal epithelium.

The most common conjunctival response to insult is inflammation, and the commonest insult is bacterial infection. Drying out of the tear secretion may make the conjunctiva injected in its own right, and may produce a fertile breeding ground for the same infections. When a normally wet membrane dries out it produces a feeling of grittiness, and not surprisingly dryness—rather like the sensation in the throat after a night spent with an open mouth. Infective conjunctivitis usually responds to intensive application of local antibiotic drops. Drainage is facilitated by *not* applying an eye pad.

Non-purulent conjunctivitis that does not respond to intensive antibiotic drop therapy can reasonably be ascribed to virus infection. The condition may be isolated or part of an epidemic shared by users of the same swimming pool. Excessive chlorination of the water to prevent such infections may produce conjunctival appearances not dissimilar from the infection they seek to prevent. As long as it is realised that any local applications will do nothing to remove the virus, emmolient lotions such as artificial tears or castor oil may soothe the patient and make them feel that something is being done.

Subconjunctival haemorrhage
No treatment is required for this condition, which may be recognised by the total obliteration of vascular markings. If recurrent and bilateral, and associated with haemorrhages elsewhere, investigation of unnatural bleeding will be indicated.

Spring catarrh

This allergic condition begins in early life and tends to improve during the mid teens. More common perhaps in those children unfortunate enough to suffer eczema and asthma, it produces giant papillae on the deep surface of the eyelids (Fig. 39), threatening the corneal surface and indeed occasionally abrading it into an ulcer.

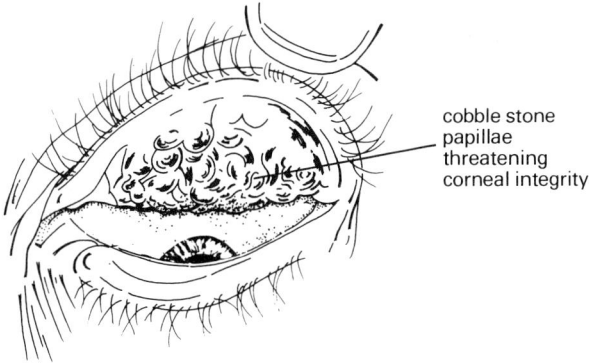

cobble stone
papillae
threatening
corneal integrity

Fig. 39 Spring catarrh
      Part of the infantile eczema-asthma syndrome. One of the exceptional conditions where hydrocortisone may be applied in the presence of a staining cornea

This is one of the few cases where corticosteroids may be used in the presence of a broken epithelium. Clearly it is potentially dangerous, but leaving the papillae to break the epithelium further might be more dangerous. It is best to leave this decision to an ophthalmologist, who has more sophisticated equipment to assess the extent of the condition, and has sufficient legal standing should the course of management not run entirely to plan.

Kerato-conjunctivitis sicca

Absent tears, more common perhaps in post-menopausal women, also dry the eyes of younger people who suffer from one of the rheumatic disorders. More recently it occurred as the result of an extreme response to one of the cardio-selective beta blocking agents (Practolol). That one sex is pre-eminently chosen to suffer the simple dry eye, is one of nature's little ironies.

Concretions

Tiny hardened calcareous deposits in the tarsal conjunctiva may fret against the cornea with obvious results. They may be scraped away with a needle before any harm is done.

THE CORNEA

The cornea is the clear curved window on the front of the eye, blending with the sclera at the corneoscleral limbus. It is transparent and avascular and convex forwards. Its various layers have been described, but deep to the anterior epithelium is Bowman's membrane—the only barrier between injury and a corneal scar. Its own blood supply is derived from the blood vessels around the limbus, and it is for this reason that any inflammation of the cornea or anything deep to it is recognised by injection of these blood vessels— circum-corneal injection.

Keratitis

Any breach of the corneal epithelium might fairly be called keratitis— whether it be due to a superficial foreign body, an abrasion or an infection. It is wise to make certain from the history whether or not something was travelling fast enough to penetrate the globe.

Herpes simplex keratitis

Though probably less common than the bacterial ulcer, this infection of the cornea by the herpes simplex virus can be a most damaging and lethal condition. Spreading from local reservoirs of infection, either a cold sore, the upper respiratory tract or indeed the conjunctiva itself, the virus settles in the corneal epithelium causing a classically branching ulcer which has given rise to its other more popular name— dendritic (Fig. 40). The pattern will be made more obvious with sodium fluorescein.

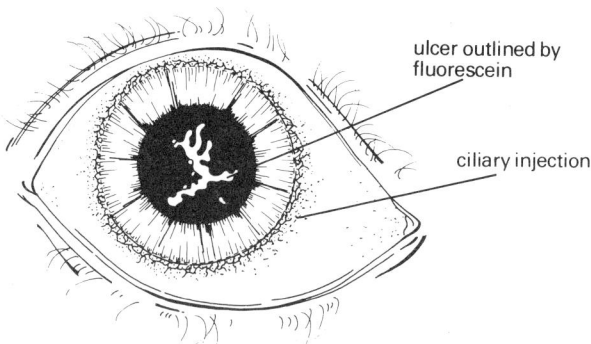

Fig. 40 Dendritic ulcer
The condition where NO form of cortisone may be applied in the presence of a staining cornea

As any other infection it may seed itself across the corneal epithelium and penetrate the stroma through Bowman's membrane.

Once it has healed, it has a permanently damaging effect on corneal sensation, diminishing the natural protection of the eye against trivial injury or recurrent infection.

Anti-viral drops may kill the virus before it damages the cornea. In hospital practice chemical cautery is perhaps more popular. Under local drop anaesthesia, a pointed orange stick dipped in absolute alcohol or phenol can be used to scrape away the infected epithelium. Atropine drops keep the pupil out of danger's way should the keratitis have become a kerato-iritis. The pain may be exquisite when the effects of the local anaesthetic have worn off.

Once the cornea has healed, the corneal sensation is unfortunately permanently diminished. As a result, the cornea has lost one of its prime defence mechanisms against recurrent invasion, and will be forever vulnerable. From time to time an allergic reaction to a virus infection produces a cloudy disc in the depths of the cornea, and a neat medical dilemma as well. Treatment of this hazy disc is corticosteroid. Treatment of the virus is anything but. Such a dilemma must be faced by the ophthalmologist alone when dilute and tentative solutions of corticosteroid might be considered.

Long standing ulcers, whatever their origin, that fail to heal, do appear from time to time. Because there is no mechanism to induce corneal healing, the only recourse is to produce circumstances in which the cornea might be allowed to heal. This is best achieved by stitching the eyelids together (tarsorrhaphy), for the eyelids may need to remain closed for some months. The cynical might sneer at this convenient concealment of medical failure. Whatever the truth in their gibes, the epithelium usually does what is expected of it.

Superficial corneal foreign bodies

Removal may be carried out under local anaesthesia, either with a moistened cotton-tipped applicator, or a broad gauged needle should the cotton tip fail. Either of these is preferable to the traditional corneal spud, as delicate as its name, which, although designed to remove foreign bodies, is much more effective at producing further corneal abrasions around an immobile fragment.

Subtarsal foreign body

The lower fornix can be easily seen when the eyelid is pulled away from the globe. The upper is not quite so easy. It can, however, be brought into view by turning the upper eyelid. This is achieved by pulling on the lashes whilst pressing a match or some similarly shaped blunt object on the skin fold at the upper margin of the tarsal plate. It is as well to warn the patient that this might be uncomfortable, because it usually is. The upper fornix can then be brought into view by pressing the lower eyelid against the globe, and any foreign body may then be brushed away with a wet pledget of cotton wool.

If a foreign body has landed on the cornea or in the conjunctival sac, it should be remembered that one might have gone through the globe as well. If any doubt exists, X-ray of the orbit is mandatory.

Corneal erosion
Recurrent breach of the corneal epithelium frequently follows injury—not least an unexpected little hand across a mother's admiring eyes. The epithelium dislodged from its connection with Bowman's membrane adheres instead overnight to the eyelid, which then rips it off in the morning. The pain is fearful, and when the patient has recovered, after a few days, the whole cycle may begin again.

The pinpoint erosions of superficial punctate keratitis following either ultra-violet burns (welder's flash or snow blindness), or in response to tear deficiency, have one thing in common with the previous condition—namely areas of broken or absent epithelium. These cannot be made to heal. They will heal only if circumstances are favourable, and in their own time. Closure of the eyelids in the first instance with micropore tape is the best way to create these favourable circumstances. Tubes and bottles may not be the best way.

Corneal lacerations
As can be guessed, the danger is of infection and damage to the delicate lens and aqueous drainage apparatus. It must be remembered that what went in might not have come out again, and a retained intra-ocular foreign body will eventually destroy the eye with infection or deposition of metallic salts throughout its vital tissues. Corneal lacerations are a perfect entry portal for infection. They are also a perfect exit portal for ocular contents should any pressure be carelessly applied to the globe. Local antibiotic drops and an eye pad are perhaps the safest first aid measures prior to hospital referral.

Corneal graft
The cornea, being free of blood vessels in its stroma, is an ideal tissue to accept donor material from sources that might not be acceptable to any other organ. The material, healthy before death, should be preferably less than 24 hours old. A disc of diseased cornea is replaced with a disc of donor cornea and stitched into position. These stitches, as foreign bodies, naturally stimulate the growth of blood vessels from the corneal limbus which, while bringing healing material, may also threaten the donor button with rejecting antibodies.

CONDITIONS THAT CROSS THE BOUNDARIES BETWEEN THE LIDS, THE CONJUNCTIVA AND THE CORNEA

Herpes Zoster ophthalmicus

This infection by the chicken-pox virus (varicella) causes vesiculation along any branch of the ophthalmic division of the trigeminal nerve (Fig. 41). These vesicles change to pustules and form thick tenacious crusts, which appear in crops and sprays over the forehead and the upper eyelids. The conjunctiva and cornea may or may not be affected, but they tend to succumb in order. Indeed the inflammation may spread deeper still, affecting the iris, and the choroid as well. The condition becomes dangerous when a corneal ulcer forms. In addition, damage to the drainage mechanism of the eye will give rise to a glaucoma,

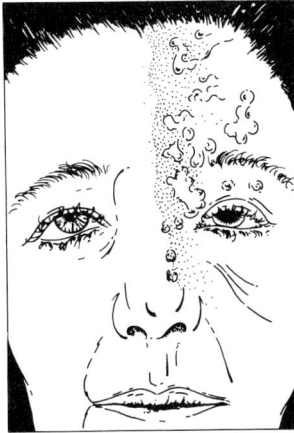

Fig. 41 Herpes zoster ophthalmicus
Dermatitis of the upper eyelid, conjunctivitis, keratitis, iritis—four red eyes all caused by the same thing and all self evident. Glaucoma secondary to the iritis is also common but not self evident

secondary to herpetic iritis which may persist when the herpetic iritis is long forgotten. Herpes Zoster is grievously painful, remaining so long after the scabs have gone. It may take three to four months to clear completely, leaving shiny thin skin where once there were pustules. Shingles elsewhere has been called 'the girdle of roses from hell'. As far as the eye is concerned, the word 'girdle' may not be appropriate but its source without doubt is. Corneal sensation is of course reduced, and so also may be its clarity.

Vesicles on the skin may be treated with a variety of soothing lotions. The conjunctivitis may be made more comfortable with local corticosteroids—another flagrant breach of the rule about cortico- steroids and broken corneal epithelium. This breach should be left to the ophthalmologist.

Trachoma

The commonest cause of blindness in the Third World is due to this infection. Ironically the infective agents (the chlamydia) do not in themselves destroy the vision. They produce a toxin which causes a lymphocytic reaction and scar formation in subepithelial areas of the conjunctiva, and eventually a dry eye. But indifference to the use of soap and water, or as is more likely, the reservation of the latter for simple survival, provides a fertile breeding ground for the secondary infections which complicate the basic disease.

Scarring will produce inevitable results. The eyelids are distorted, the tear inflow blocked, the cornea infiltrated with blood vessels.

Ideally management should start with prevention, education, the provision of public health facilities, and the elimination of filth.

Tetracycline ointment used over several months deals with the active infection. The distorted lids require surgery to reduce distortion, to turn the lashes outwards, and to reconstruct the conjunctival sac. Corneal opacities may respond to corneal grafting if the cornea is not riddled with blood borne, rejecting antibodies. Artificial tears will in some way restore the natural moistened state of the conjunctival membrane.

Given the scale of this problem it is evident that most patients visually handicapped in its middle stages, will never have the opportunity of such benefits. Those in its later stages could not make use of the benefits were they offered.

Pterygium

This degenerative accumulation of tissue in the deep layers of the conjunctiva occurs along the line of the opening eyelids. More common perhaps in Europeans living in tropical exile, the condition is benign until it threatens to move across the cornea. Adopting the form of a wing, hence its name, it may relentlessly advance over the cornea from one side to the other, trailing a scar across the pupil line (Fig. 42).

They are evident in portraits of Admiral Nelson of Trafalgar fame. Indeed it is likely that one eye was not sightless at all as a result of injury. Rather, a combination of pterygium and presbyopia did more harm to both eyes than did the French guns to one.

Early excision will intercept the scar before it has ravaged the cornea. Excision however would not be required for pinguecula—a flabby yellow nodule which occupies the same areas of the conjunctiva but never threatens to cross the corneal frontier.

Episcleritis

A painful inflammatory nodule, it has the same mysterious origins as

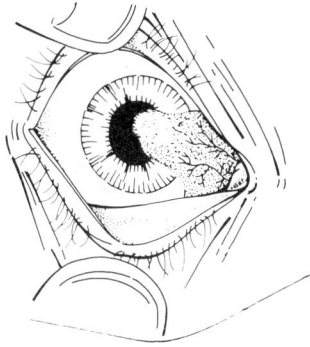

Fig. 42 Pterygium
A wing like growth which threatens corneal clarity. It should be excised when it is still threatening and not when it has reached this stage

pterygium from those tissues that lie between the conjunctiva and the sclera (Fig. 43). However there the similarity ends.

It is independent of climate, is found anywhere but the cornea, and does not figure at all in naval portraiture. It could be that its transience defeated attempts by artists to capture it on canvas. It is also possible that the general discomfort would have blunted the obligatory bold stare into posterity—which is better served nowadays by intensive corticosteroid drops, that clear away the episcleritis without trace.

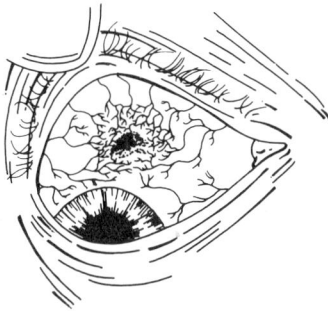

Fig. 43 Episcleritis
A painful red nodule on the sclera. The cornea and pupil are normal

Rosacea

This metabolic disturbance, which produces blotchy inflammation over the cheeks and nose, may also affect the eyes, producing the same blotchy inflammation in the conjunctiva and tongue-shaped inflammatory advances across the cornea itself. The local treatment can be worked out from what has been said before. Clearly it should be started before corneal scars have diminished the vision and made drop therapy useless.

The systemic aspects in recent years have apparently responded to long term low dosage of Tetracycline tablets. A total ban on alcohol, hot foods and other pleasing diversions has also been recommended, although there is no record that colonial administrators sustained on a diet of burra pegs and fierce curries had a higher reputation for blotchy faces than their more abstemious counterparts at home.

CONTACT LENSES

Contact lenses are foreign bodies applied to the cornea in the hope that visual improvement or emotional relief from discarding spectacles will compensate for the insult to the eye of their application. Made from a variety of synthetic transparent materials of differing physical attributes, they are accepted by the eye only in the presence of a normal fluid exchange across the corneal surface and an adequate supply of tears.

These conditions are not always met. Fluid balance throughout the body fluctuates as the normal hormonal cycles fluctuate, and when these cycles are further unbalanced by the contraceptive pill, pregnancy or impending abortion, intolerance of contact lenses may be the first indication. Should the tear secretion decline below a certain critical level, then this intolerance becomes permanent.

Even healthy eyes have their problems. Coarsely fitted lenses depriving the anterior corneal surface of oxygen will cause a hazy oedema of the epithelium. Overwearing of well fitted lenses will produce the same result, and if carried to foolish lengths, may induce the growth of superficial new vessels around the corneoscleral limbus—presumably to make up the oxygen normally supplied by the tears.

With this baleful array of hazards it is a wonder that people wear contact lenses at all. They do so for a variety of reasons. Vanity and cosmetic satisfaction can lead to a tolerance of the most appalling discomforts, and most contact lenses are worn for these reasons. However there can be no doubt that eyes with extreme refractive errors see more effectively with such lenses than they do with standard glasses. The visual field enlarges when unhampered by thick spectacle frames, and the distorting periphery of a thick lens is not used when a lens of equivalent strength is placed upon the eye. Central vision also sharpens, because contact with the eye is a much more natural optical arrangement than glasses in a frame. The pity is that it is not a more natural corneal arrangement.

Such lenses have their uses for medical reasons. Unilateral aphakics who have normal vision in the other eye may regain binocular function when a contact lens comes near to restoring the optical balance of the eye to what it was before the cataract was removed.

An abnormal curvature of the cornea (keratoconus) not only induces myopia, but also thin opaque corneal stroma at the summit of the cone. A judiciously designed lens may not only prevent this disaster, but may improve the vision as well and delay the need for corneal grafting. When corneal ulcers refuse to heal, stitching the eyelids together (tarsorrhaphy) is not always acceptable, especially in an only eye. A contact lens can be applied as a bandage to allow the corneal epithelium to regenerate without external disturbance. The lids stay open. The patient may continue to see, and the sceptical will also see that covering the cornea is not just a device to conceal therapeutic defeat.

Contact lens wearers complain from time to time of irritable eyes. This is not surprising as the potential cause has been applied by themselves. Corneal abrasions, erosions, infections and frank assault from trying to remove a contact lens that may not be in position, are all ways in which this may happen. More common still is a grumbling conjunctivitis caused by simple intolerance to the lens material, or allergy to the endless variety of solutions available for them to steep in. The routine examination ritual will show which part of the external eye has been damaged, and most symptoms will clear away when the lens is taken out. Most symptoms will stay away if the lens is kept out, at least until all the signs and any doubts over the suitability of the lens have cleared away as well.

7

The red eye

Before we can call an eye abnormal and red, we must first define what we mean by normal and white. Such a definition is based on the conjunctival appearances which vary on their position. To begin with we have the sclera seen as an egg shell white through the translucent vascular conjunctiva. The scleral dominance fades as the conjunctiva folds away into the fornix, and then towards the front again, where it becomes pinker and pinker, until arriving at the deep surface of the lids it has become almost red.

So much for the normal; there is barely more to the abnormal, for there are only three causes of inflammation that can be called serious, and they all share one major feature.

The major three—*keratitis, iritis* and *acute glaucoma*—dilate many vessels within the eyeball itself, but only those around the corneoscleral limbus are readily visible. This circumcorneal or ciliary injection is the warning sign of an eye in serious danger. All other conditions, no matter what their cause, demonstrate their indifference to these vessels by leaving a circle of pallor around the corneoscleral limbus. Now no textbook is considered complete unless it attempts to distinguish at length every cause of the red eye from every other cause, but in fact, the problem is not quite as complicated as it seems, hence the brevity of this chapter.

There is only one decision to make about a red eye. Is it one of the major three or is it not? If it is, then examination of the eye carried out in the same way every time will indicate which of the major three it is every time.

KERATITIS (Fig. 44)

In addition to pain, redness and watering, the patient will admit to loss of central vision. He may admit to a previous attack, and if he admits to several previous attacks he could conceivably disclose what his previous treatment was as well. Indeed he could possibly have already started it.

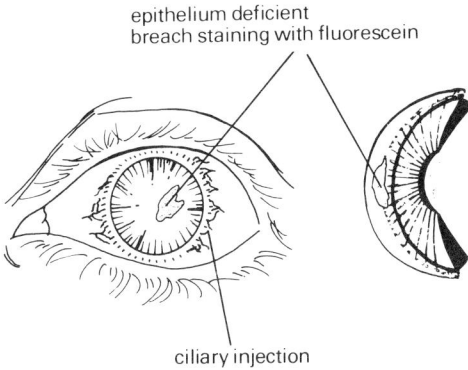

Fig. 44 Keratitis
    One of the three major red eyes; the cornea stains with fluorescein, and is seen to more clearly when brought close with a small convex lens

Reduction of central *vision* will depend on the actual position of the ulcer. The field will be unaffected.

The *corneal lustre* will be lost, and the exact area of deficient corneal epithelium can be demonstrated with sodium fluorescein.

A normal *pupil* is common in keratitis, unless an associated iritis has already stuck it to the lens. An old bottle of Atropine resurrected from the medicine cupboard along with all the other drops might have had its effect also—dilating those parts of the pupil still mobile.

The *anterior* chamber of both eyes will be deep.

IRITIS (Fig. 45)

The complaints may be very much the same as keratitis, with the addition of floaters of inflammatory debris, exuded from the iris vessels and dancing across the visual line. Surface pain also will be perhaps rather less, because the lid is not blinking over a damaged cornea. Deep pain induced by light however will be rather more.

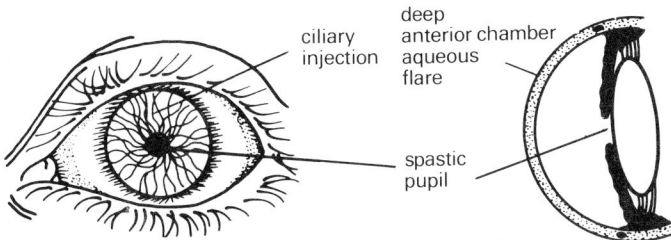

Fig. 45 Iritis
    One of the three major red eyes; the cornea is normal and the pupil possibly spastic; flare and keratic precipitates are more obvious when brought close with a small convex lens

Central *vision* can be anything from normal downwards, depending on previous damage or the severity of the present attack. The field is generally unaffected.

A clear *corneal surface* is usual, but deposits of inflammatory material (keratic precipitates) may be detected on the deep surface of the cornea with a magnifying lens.

A spastic *pupil* is common, unless distorted by previous adhesions or dilated with an old bottle of Atropine in anticipation of the same treatment again.

The *anterior chamber* in both eyes will be deep and there will be aqueous flare.

ACUTE GLAUCOMA (Fig. 46)

The evident distress of the patient will probably cut short the tell-tale story of haloes, frontal headache and transient attacks of blurred vision in the evening.

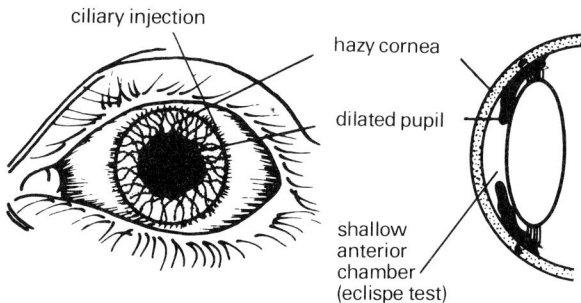

Fig. 46 Acute glaucoma
One of the three major red eyes; the cornea is hazy, the pupil fixed and dilated, the anterior chamber shallow on both sides (Eclipse test)

Central *vision* will be grievously affected, and the patient too disturbed to attend to hands flapping in his visual field.

A steamy oedematous *cornea* almost obscuring the deeper signs, is classic.

The *pupil*, however, will be seen to be fixed and dilated.

If the *anterior* chamber be obscured on the affected side, an eclipse test on the follow eye will leave the iris remote from the light in shadow—the hallmark of the shallow fronted eye.

The affected eye will be rock hard. It will also be acutely tender.

Once we can recognise when an eye is inflamed by one of these major three, we will also be in a position to recognise when it is not. *As a general rule the less dangerous a red eye might be, the more alarming it will appear.* Subconjunctival haemorrhage and conjunctivitis can both seem frightful, and if the cardinal signs of the cornea and the pupil are neglected in favour of the overall impression, then they may be given a greater significance than they deserve. They may even give a spurious attraction to the alternative but lethal subdivision of inflamed eyes into those that seem to improve with corticosteroids and those that do not. Although common, this subdivision is unacceptable.

Of the three major causes of a red eye, keratitis has signs in the cornea. Acute glaucoma has signs in the cornea, the anterior chamber depth and the pupil. Iritis may have only ciliary injection to mark it off from other lesser causes of a red eye. Only very close examination will reveal signs on the deep surface of the cornea, and in a first attack the spastic pupil may be not very different from its fellow on the other side. The special rule is to use the same examination ritual every time, and not to suspend our clinical judgement just because the redness happens to be in the eye and not somewhere else.

8

When the lacrimal drainage goes wrong

The eyes could not survive without tears, yet when the lacrimal system is upset, it is watering that people complain about most bitterly. Dryness of the eye, on the other hand, with its associated complications are inventively ascribed to a variety of causes and not connected in any way with the lacrimal apparatus. A significant and common cause of recurrent irritation, it opens the eye to all manner of infections which flourish on the unhealthy conjunctiva (Fig. 47).

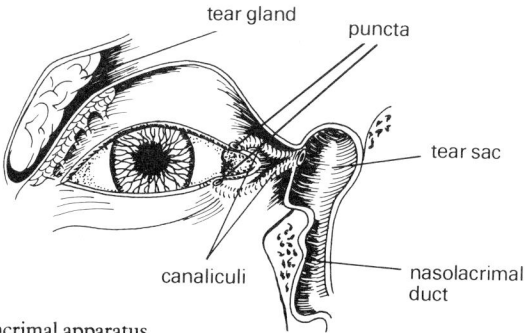

Fig. 47 The lacrimal apparatus
A dry eye is more common than a watering one. Poorly positioned puncta are a commoner cause of a watering eye than is a blocked nasolacrimal duct

There are two basic kinds of tear flow. Firstly, the basal production which is necessary to keep the conjunctival 'synovial' membrane healthy. The second is the reflex flood in response to some disturbance—like a foreign body or a finger in the eye.

If the basal flow be diminished the ensuing grittiness may stimulate the remaining glandular cells into activity. The eye sometimes responds to tear deficiency paradoxically by watering.

EPIPHORA

This is the name given to any condition where tears appear on the wrong side of the eyelids. It may follow excessive production or diminished drainage.

Excess production

Although quoted in most text books as being the early sign of a lacrimal gland tumour, excess tears are almost invariably the result of irritation of some kind or another.

Deficient drainage

The drainage system from the eyelids to the nose depends not only on patency but on snug contact between the eyelid and the eyeball. Ill fitting lids can cause apparent lacrimal problems by exposure of the eyeball and by separating the tear puncta from the globe.

Blockage of tear ducts

Interference with the tear flow anywhere along the line of drainage will result in epiphora with an excess of tears. Should these tears become totally stagnant then they may well become infected as well.

Blockage in the canaliculus is particularly difficult to treat. The canaliculi are so fine that surgery upon them may increase rather than decrease the obstruction.

The great reservoir for tears is the lacrimal sac which may explode into a lacrimal abscess, classically recognised as an angry red swelling between the nose and the medial canthus. Pressure on the tear sac may produce pus at the lacrimal puncta.

In children, a membrane, at the lower end of the nasal lacrimal duct occasionally remains imperforate. It is possible to clear this membrane by probing the duct under general anaesthesia. However in the absence of lacrimal sac infection there is much to be said for waiting in the hope that simple growth will produce the necessary opening. Lacrimal passages are very delicate, and a coarsely handled probe may turn a temporary blockage into a permanent one.

Blockage in adults is a common occurrence in our temperate climate, and as often as not, related to chronic nasal catarrh. If surgery be deemed necessary it involves cracking a hole in the bone between the lacrimal fossa and the nasal cavity. A junction is then effected between the lacrimal sac and the nasal mucosa. Closure of this junction is not infrequent, as the body does not tolerate abnormal apertures.

It is as well to ask patients if their symptoms are bad enough to make them want an operation. Not infrequently the threat of such a procedure makes the symptoms suddenly more tolerable than they appeared to be, at the start of the interview.

This tolerance can be increased by applying local astringents, like drops containing zinc sulphate, to the eye. Constricting drops in the nostril may constrict the lining at the lower end of the duct, just enough to improve the symptoms beyond the critical level of awareness.

Trauma

Rupture of the canaliculus in the lower lid is a common windscreen injury. It is vital to secure the torn ends immediately, arranging them around a silicone rubber tube where hopefully they will heal without stricture. The tube may have to be left in place for six months.

Failure produces intractable watering that defeats the ingenuity of the surgeon, the tolerance of the patient, and may produce a mountain of legal and insurance reports.

It must not be assumed therefore that all watering is due to blockage along the nasolacrimal duct. If surgery is not contemplated, and there is no evidence of lacrimal sac infection then there is nothing to be gained by invading the ducts with a coarse and possibly infected probe.

If the patient did not start off with a lacrimal sac infection, it is not inconceivable that he could end up with it. Simple drops to the eye and nostril are the first move. Threat of surgery is the second, and an actual operation may well be the start of a series.

9

Haemorrhages and Exudates

HAEMORRHAGE

Bleeding in the eye occurs for the same reasons as bleeding elsewhere. But haemorrhage joins with exudates as an obscure ocular duo that flourishes outside the confines of general pathology. Indeed a recent colour plate publication showed a boomerang-shaped retinal haemorrhage with the caption 'Lymphatic leukaemia'—as though myeloid leukaemia might present with something different but equally diagnostic. It was of course diagnostic of neither, indicating only blood, the presence of which had to be explained by the routine investigations for bleeding.

The simpler approach is to consider first of all why haemorrhage occurs, and secondly where. In general terms abnormal bleeding results from one of three basic reasons:

1. Abnormalities of the blood vessel.
2. Abnormalities of the blood.
3. Abnormalities of the blood pressure.

Most commonly the blood vessels suffer from some systemic disease, such as diabetes or hypertension. The same systemic conditions can favour the existence of back pressure along the veins resulting in acute venous blockage, aptly named the stormy sunset retina.

Violence or an unprovoked injury—for example a retinal tear leading to a retinal detachment—can produce haemorrhage as well.

Spontaneous tissue change, whether in the form of tumour necrosis or macular degeneration likewise produces leakage from otherwise normal vessels.

Retinal ischaemia, due either to diabetes or hypertension, or when the cause is unknown—'Eales' disease'—produces fragile new vessels in the retina. In the eye the one feature these vessels share above all others is their fragility. They form to bring oxygen and all they bring is blood, which does not remain within them.

The clotting mechanisms seem an ever-changing tangle of strangely named clotting factors and platelets. Spontaneous abnormal bleeding follows disorders of either, be they hereditary or one of the blood dyscrasias.

Hypertension has many causes and its effect on the eye depends on its speed of onset and degree, ranging from fine flecks on the retina to a black vitreous which allows no view of the retina at all.

Haemorrhages vary in shape depending upon their position, and from these variations we can pick up clues, if not to a diagnosis, at least to a sensible plan of investigation.

Haemorrhages deep in the retina are limited in shape by the close packing of retinal tissue and are generally round. These are most common in diabetes.

As they approach nearer to the surface of the retina the looser arrangement of nerve fibres allows greater scope for spread and surface haemorrhages on the retina tend to take on a spray pattern along the line of the retinal fibres. They are a feature of hypertension.

As the tendency becomes more severe blood may burst from the retina into the vitreous. On the way it may form a fluid level before the retina, resulting in a haemorrhage shaped like a D on its side. Since most people spend much of their lives vertical the sharp edge of the D will also be pointing upwards.

Within the vitreous proper there are no constraints on its shape, and blood may float and coil through the cavity, modified only in its movements by the viscosity of the vitreous and in its abundance by the precipitating disaster.

A retinal tear on its way to a retinal detachment may present such a haemorrhage. So may hitherto unsuspected diabetes in the elderly.

Macular degeneration

Local haemorrhage at the posterior pole of the eye, although possibly related to hypertension, may be part of a spontaneous degeneration of the macula.

Hyphaema

Intra-ocular blood does not always occupy the posterior cavity of the eye. It can be found in the anterior chamber between the iris and the cornea, again with a fluid level (Fig. 48). Usually the result of trauma, it may also occur spontaneously as a result of one of the bleeding disorders.

This is thus the extent of intra-ocular haemorrhage. *Retinal detachment, macular degeneration* and *Eales's disease* are the only conditions that occur because they happen to be inside the eye. Even they have a basis in general pathology along with the rest. Vitreal

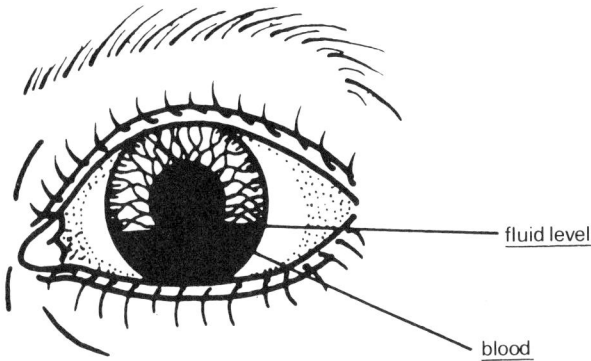

Fig. 48 Hyphaema
A blow sufficient to cause this may cause other things as well (see Fig. 88)

haemorrhage is more dangerous because it stimulates a fibrotic reaction within the vitreal cavity itself. Fibrosis in common with scars anywhere will result in contracting bands which, if attached to the retina, will shrink, pulling the vision with it.

Blood entirely filling the anterior chamber may stain the cornea if under pressure for long.

All other haemorrhages will affect the eye according to their position, and although they may disperse spontaneously after a few months or even years, especially if the underlying cause be removed, they may still leave permanent damage behind.

A simple level of investigation should include measurement of the blood pressure, examination of the urine for sugar and protein, and a full blood count. A search for the more exotic clotting problems rarely comes into the picture for the patient has usually got into the clutches of a haematologist long before ophthalmic haemorrhages demand the attention of yet another specialist.

EXUDATES

The second partner of our duo of signs—exudates—is another feature hesitantly mentioned when an instant fundal opinion is demanded.

There are two kinds of exudates—hard and soft—although, this is a visual distinction, for both would disintegrate under the fingers.

Hard exudates

These are of fatty origin lying at various depths in the retina. Whether from local degeneration of retinal nervous tissue or whether a product of fatty leakage, is a moot point. The colour shades from yellow to waxy white, but all of them, if left for any length of time, will destroy the overlying retina.

The common general conditions that give rise to hard exudates are diabetes and hypertension. Both may damage central vision, the former with random shapeless exudates, the latter with a star pattern tracing the normal macular anatomy in fat.

Other causes of hard exudates are much more rare. Clearly any local condition of the small blood vessels can give rise to exudates. These can occur in little circles around diabetic capillary malformations.

More rarely still, exudates may fill the entire posterior pole, elevating the retina in front of them. The cause is a bizarre conglomeration of abnormal vessels, usually in the periphery of one eye of young males. The explanation sadly still lurks undetected behind the eponym Coats' disease.

Macular degeneration
Haemorrhage does not have a monopoly on the macula. Exudates too may demonstrate declining function in old people. Indeed they may both appear together.

Soft exudates
Strictly speaking these are not exudates at all. They resemble little fluffy patches of cotton wool. They are transient and scattered, and can be thought of as retinal infarcts, which block from view the normal red choroidal pattern. Although their exact pathological nature is a source of lively disagreement, they can be regarded as an index of severe underlying vascular disease, and must always worsen the long term prognosis of anyone unfortunate enough to have them.

Diabetes and hypertension again head the list of likely causes. Thereafter we must consider disorders of the blood vessels, like the so-called collagen diseases, dubbed by an eminent pathologist 'the call again diseases'. Any blood disorder that gives rise to anaemia, be it simple iron deficiency or leukaemia, can give rise to soft exudates.

Acute closure of the central retinal artery might be considered a giant cotton wool spot, clouding the entire retina and obscuring the choroid, except at the central area of the retina—the macula—where the retina is too thin to hide the choroidal redness. This is the familiar cherry red spot associated with total loss of light perception.

Chorioretinitis
Active inflammation of the choroid and retina, whatever the cause, gives rise to a fluffy soft patch in the retina. The diagnosis will be suggested by the overlying vitreous haze, which must first be distinguished from faulty ophthalmoscopy.

Healed focal chorioretinitis (Fig. 49) looks very much like a hard exudate. The clue to its origin lies in the other signs of inflammation that have given rise to it. Any inflammatory episode in the retina and choroid disturb the pigment epithelium, which forms a black border of heaped pigment around a hard white lesion, where the sclera is visible through a window of deficient pigment.

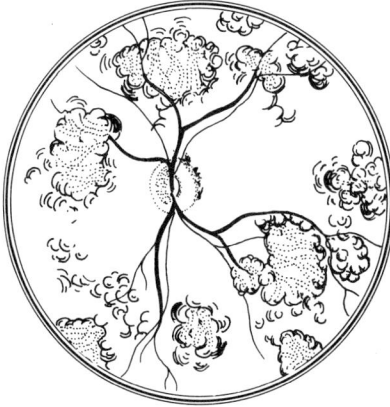

Fig. 49 Scars of healed chorio-retinitis
A breach of the treaty between the ocular layers—atrophy of the neural retina, pigment retina and much of the choroid exposes bare sclera with the odd choroidal vessel and pigment clumps remaining as evidence of the conflict

10

Diabetes and the eye

Diabetes is one of the most common causes of blindness in Western countries today. In the young, its major complication—retinopathy— begins some 15 years after the onset of the disease, but there is no doubt that this time lapse can be extended by careful diabetic control.

Maturity onset diabetics, on the contrary, may be quite unaware of their metabolic problems until a sudden vitreal haemorrhage initiates a series of medical investigations that seem bafflingly remote from the eye.

It is impossible to get any measure of the incidence of this condition, but it is wise to assume that all diabetics are liable. It is therefore the obligation of all medical practitioners who undertake the care of a diabetic to examine both fundi under mydriasis every year, shortening the period to six months should retinopathy be discovered. Failure to do so constitutes neglect.

The diabetic retina has come in for its fair share of numerical gradings but the sum of such efforts is to put a number on our ignorance and call it science. We also tend to forget what the numbers mean.

Perhaps it is better to remember that diabetic retinal changes occur from one basic lesion in the walls of the small blood vessels— microangiopathy. This process affects blood vessels all over the body, but only in the eye is its evil so evident.

Local swellings in these small vessels give rise to microaneurysms, seen as rounded red blobs scattered throughout the fundus.

Such vessels have a tendency to leak both blood and fat into the retina. Haemorrhages appear of course to be red in colour, the shape and distribution dictated by their position. Deep haemorrhages appear round, surface haemorrhages appear flame-shaped. Pre-retinal haemorrhages take on a fluid level, and vitreous haemorrhages flood through the vitreal cavity (Fig. 50).

Fatty leakage results in hard exudates, usually around the macula. Incompetence of these retinal vessels results in oxygen deprivation. Sudden closure gives rise to an acute retinal infarct—a cotton wool spot that hides the normal choroidal pattern from view.

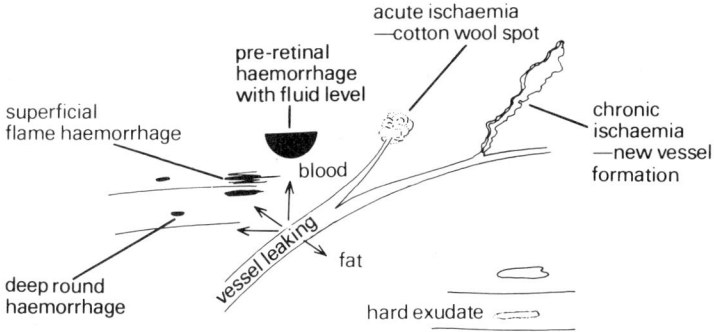

Fig. 50 Diabetic micro-angiopathy
The process behind what we call diabetic retinopathy

More leisurely blockage causes hypoxia. Poorly fed retinal tissue then in search of more oxygen creates new blood vessels in the hope of supplying this want. However, instead of oxygen the retina gets blood, because these vessels have a tendency to spontaneous rupture—a tendency encouraged by hypertension and anything leading to abnormal rises in blood pressure.

Distortion and dilatation of the retinal veins can be taken as a reliable sign of an unhealthy retinal circulation.

The old distinction between background retinopathy and proliferative retinopathy is now questioned. One must assume that all forms of retinopathy, no matter how bland they look, are capable of turning on the offensive. This offensive takes two forms. The first is obliteration of central vision due to macular hard exudates, especially in older diabetes.

The second and perhaps more common, is the cycle of new blood vessel and vitreal bleeding followed by fibrosis and traction retinal detachment (Fig. 51). This cycle can lead to total blindness.

Although retinopathy dominates the picture, it is not the whole story. Diabetic eyes under surgery bleed where others would not, and tend to respond with greater post-operative inflammation than others might. New vessel formation is not confined to the retina. It can creep over the iris and produce a catastrophic blockage to aqueous flow and cause a particularly intractable form of secondary glaucoma. Cataract at an earlier stage than normal completes this array of disaster.

MANAGEMENT

Fatty macular exudates, once they have developed, leave behind

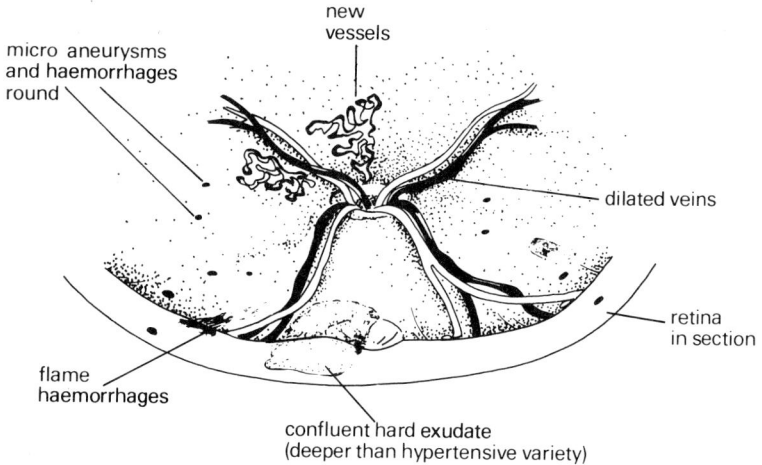

Fig. 51 Diabetic retinopathy
Related to duration and poor control

permanent visual damage. Treatment therefore starts with recognition of those eyes at risk, followed by Clofibrate to reduce the level of blood lipids. Despite the question mark over the life shortening qualities of Clofibrate the drug must surely be justified to preserve the macular function of patients whose life expectancy is, alas, shortened anyway.

The bleeding tendency recognised by an abundance of retinal haemorrhage, soft exudates and above all new blood vessel formation, especially on the optic disc, is an indication for light coagulation.

Large areas of the retina have to be destroyed by the Xenon light coagulator, or more fashionably by the Argon Laser (Fig. 52). The theoretical basis is that such destruction of the retina leaves the existing blood supply in balance with the oxygen requirements of the remaining retina, thus removing the stimulus to new vessel formation. Although this approach seems coarse, the visual results may be remarkable, and the absence of visual defect even more so.

In some healthy young diabetics (under the age of 35) complete destruction of the pituitary gland is required because the retinopathy breaks out of control despite widespread light coagulation. This is a last resort, not without its surgical complications, and it should be limited to patients who are equipped mentally to deal with the choice before them.

Effective control of retinopathy usually averts the danger of secondary glaucoma. But once that has occurred, the choices of treatment are limited. All the standard measures for glaucoma fail, and drainage operations can be carried out only if the bleeding

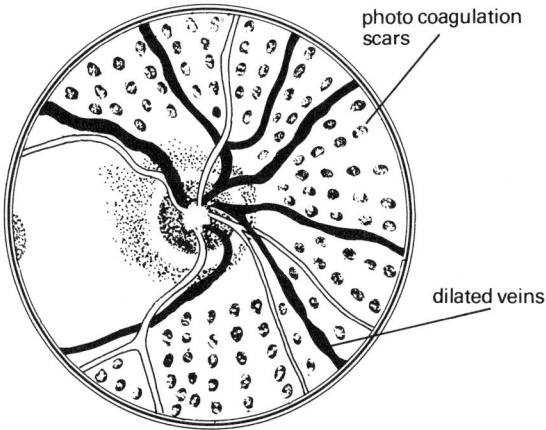

photo coagulation
scars

dilated veins

Fig. 52 Diabetic retinopathy treated with the argon laser
An iatrogenic healed chorioretinitis

tendency is curbed prior to surgery. It is conceivable that Laser photocoagulation could achieve this last condition, but all the complications of standard glaucoma surgery are multiplied because the diabetic eye does not tolerate surgery lightly.

Obliteration of the ciliary body with diathermy or freezing, if carried out gently, will not work. Carried out brutally it may be too successful and will eliminate the glaucoma, the aqueous secretion, the transparency of the transparent tissues, and eventually all resemblance to an eye as well. To be fair, though, the underlying condition can in the end achieve very much the same thing. It may be a kindness to the patient to accept the signs as inevitable and reduce his awareness of the symptoms with a retrobulbar injection of absolute alcohol.

Ophthalmologists tend to see the unpleasant face of diabetes, but none the less there are some generally unpalatable facts about the disease that make it easier to talk about only when they affect other people. And not always then, for one of the complications of treatment is depression in the ophthalmologist involved.

When one eye is blind from diabetic retinopathy the chances are that the second eye will follow in about eighteen months. When both eyes are blind, the life expectancy is limited to an average of eight years. This frightful statistic became evident only when it was realised that blind diabetics rarely returned for a second guide dog.

11

Hypertension and the eye

The response of the eye to hypertension, like so much else can be made incomprehensible if desired over several chapters. Yet predictably enough the whole matter can be reduced to three simple elements.

1. *The state of the blood vessels before the onset of hypertension.*
2. *The rate of hypertensive change.*
3. *The extent of hypertensive change.*

The state of the blood vessels
In the childhood eye, the retinal venules and the arterioles are of equal width. Both are well endowed with elastic tissue and the arterioles also with muscle. They glisten regularly in the light of an ophthalmoscope.

As the blood pressure pulses normally over the years, the elastic and muscles are replaced by fibrous material which dulls the glistening arteriolar reflex.

The calibre of the arterioles becomes reduced slightly, and the shifting highlights of the young retina give way to a dry coarse mottling. When the age of decline arrives, these fibrotic changes may, without offence, be given the name *involutionary sclerosis*.

The fundamental point is that the retinal vessels of a young eye full of elastic tissue and muscle, when faced with hypertension, will behave very differently from the vessels of an older eye which are already rigid with fibrosis (Fig. 53).

THE RATE AND EXTENT OF HYPERTENSIVE CHANGE

Hypertension arrives in different ways. It may come slowly and rise but moderately. It may come swiftly and reach unreadable levels.

Gradual rise of blood pressure (less than 200/120 mm Hg)

The ageing eye
The changes mentioned under involutionary sclerosis become exag-

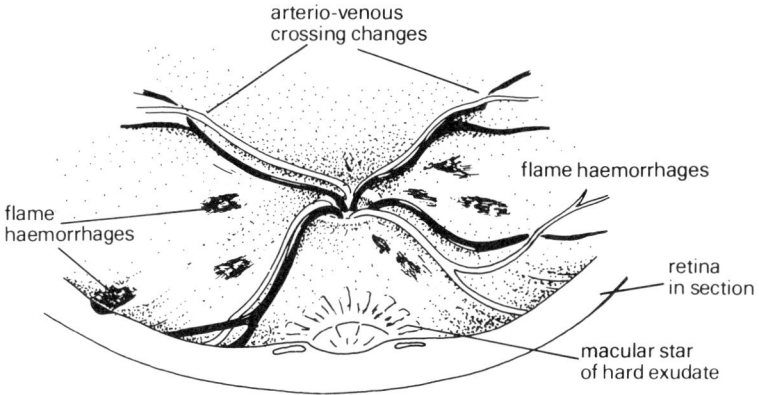

Fig. 53 Hypertensive retinopathy
Only the arterio-venous crossing changes and the macular star are unique to hypertension

gerated. Any remaining arteriolar muscle goes into spasm, and the fibrosed stems remain very much as they were, or even dilate somewhat. This explains the well known arteriolar calibre variation.

The traditional copper and silver wiring, accorded such importance in successive generations of textbooks, are merely a reflexion of the early primitive ophthalmoscope or of failing batteries in the more modern instruments. These changes are of little value and can be of interest only to students of minutiae.

Changes now develop at the arterio-venous crossings. These follow thickening of the arteriole, obvious where it crosses over or under a vein and gives the illusion of actual compression. The arterio-venous crossing change can be taken as the point where involutionary sclerosis becomes a pathological sign of hypertension. Its significance increases with distance from the disc.

The youthful eye
Such eyes will develop involutionary sclerosis which, although physiological at 60 is pathological at 20. They will then go on to develop the arterio-venous crossing change.

Both the young and the old eyes will then develop flame haemorrhages in the surface layers of the retina and hard exudates at the macula, with associated loss of central vision.

Rapid rise in hypertension (200/120 mm of mercury)

The ageing eye
All the changes described above will develop,—but more quickly.

There is no doubt that the presence of involutionary sclerosis protects the actual vessels against the more savage effects of severe hypertension.

The youthful eye
These eyes suffer grievously. The entire wall of the arteriole goes into spasm recognised by severe and regular attenuation, as a prelude to retinal necrosis. The retina becomes oedematous, and it is in this age of patient that the blood pressure reading usually goes off the scale.

Both young and old eyes may develop cotton wool spots due to small retinal infarcts. Haemorrhages present in simple hypertension will, of course, become more florid and may indeed burst into the vitreal cavity.

The optic disc becomes swollen—papilloedema (malignant hypertension).

Grading
As with diabetic retinopathy, there has been a fashion to split hypertension into numbered categories. This is just a question of adding a number to what is already perfectly simple to describe. Subsequent erudite exchanges on the matter rather lose their value if decisions taken on one grading actually refer to another.

Complications

Occlusion of the central retinal artery
Such a calamity results in a total retinal infarction. The ophthalmic appearance is that of a giant cotton wool spot (Fig. 54).

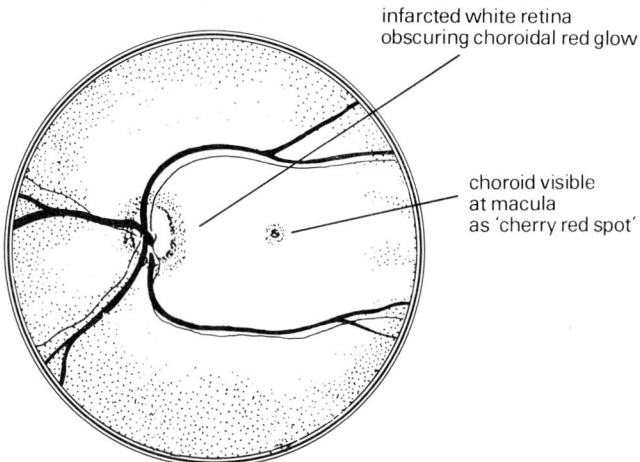

infarcted white retina
obscuring choroidal red glow

choroid visible
at macula
as 'cherry red spot'

Fig. 54 Occlusion of the central retinal artery

Occlusion of the central retinal vein

The retina is oedematous and haemorrhagic. The disc is swollen, the vision severely impaired, and the ophthalmoscopic picture that of a stormy sunset retina (Fig. 55A & B). Such eyes are ischaemic and always prone to develop new blood vessels, wherever the oxygen needs are greatest as they do in diabetic eyes.

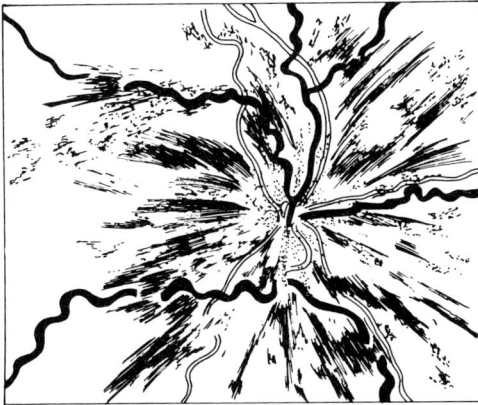

Fig. 55A Occlusion of the central retinal vein—the 'stormy sunset'
More common in patients with hypertension and chronic simple glaucoma

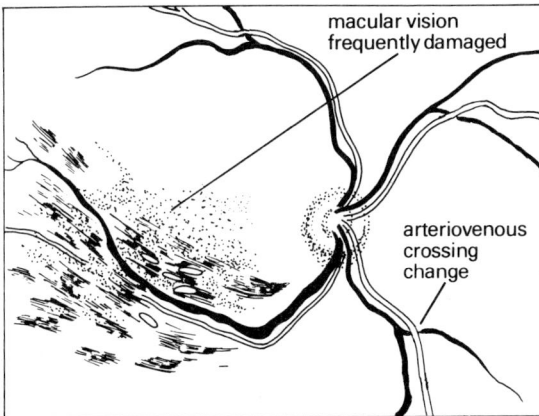

Fig. 55B Occlusion of a branch of the central retinal vein
May damage central vision and little else

In the months following central retinal vein occlusion, while the visual acuity improves, the oxygen supply to the drainage angle apparently does not. As the new blood vessels develop in the anterior chamber, the eye succumbs to the 'hundred day' glaucoma—rather like Napoleon's last throw from Elba to Waterloo—starting with hope and ending with blood.

Vitreal haemorrhage
Fragile capillaries rupturing into the vitreal cavity may clear briefly, to reveal no actual sources of bleeding, before a fresh flood of haemorrhage obscures the fundus again.

Treatment
There are one or two simple principles. Young patients may have some recognisable cause for their hypertension, which can be removed with total recovery.

The problem starts in the elderly, who may well be used to their level of blood pressure, where overkeen reduction might turn a simple ophthalmoscopic observation into a genuine disability. The presence of even one cotton wool spot means the vascular tree is already beyond repair. In general terms the more pronounced the arterio-venous crossing change the less likely is treatment to be successful.

It is too late to remove macular exudates once they have formed. Their existence should be forestalled.

The ophthalmologist can do little to treat any resultant visual loss. All he can do is warn the physician what his findings imply.

12

The lens

The crystalline lens has one basic response to insult. It becomes opaque. Different degrees of disturbance cause different degrees of opacity, but whatever their degree we call them all cataract, preferably softening the word, for most people have a mortal dread of the name.

Aetiology
The following list need not be memorised. It merely demonstrates that ocular tissues are vulnerable to the same conditions that may damage tissues elsewhere in the body. It is not limited to the eye and will not be repeated.

Congenital
Maternal infection with for example German Measles (rubella) during the first trimester of pregnancy is most likely to damage the developing lens.

Hereditary
There may be a familial tendency to cataract formation in one or both eyes at an early stage.

Traumatic
Blunt injuries and penetrating injuries, of which intra-ocular surgery for glaucoma is an example, may disturb the fluids around the lens sufficiently to disturb the lens itself. Actual rupture of the lens capsule with windscreen glass or a metallic foreign body rapidly produces a dense cataract.

Inflammation
Long standing iritis may poison the aqueous around the lens.

Neoplasia
No tumour arises directly from the lens, but rarely ciliary body tumours adjacent to the lens might conceivably affect its function.

Metabolic

The fluctuating sugar levels of diabetes exert a baneful influence across the lens capsule, resulting in diminished clarity of the lens at an age earlier than one might expect. This parallels the diabetic influence all over the body.

Radiation

All forms of ionising radiation must be regarded as harmful. Prolonged exposure to infra-red light is also a classic cause of cataract. The traditional example is the occupation of glass blower inflating his molten creations in front of his nose. Fat dogs whose only exercise is to blink their eyelids from time to time before a grate full of blazing logs suffer the same condition.

Toxic

Long term administration of corticosteroids is traditionally associated with changes in the lens.

Degeneration

By far the commonest form of cataract is the senile variety. However progressive myopia can produce changes in the lens as well.

Vascular

There is no recognised association between vascular disorders and cataract.

Pathology

Various changes take place within the lens substance. First of all an increase in water content gives way finally to dehydration. Changes in the lens proteins and electrolytes have also been recorded, but in too disconnected a fashion to be turned into a therapeutic arrest of cataract formation. Needless to say this has not dissuaded mountebanks from pedalling a variety of nostrums to produce such an arrest, some based on fancy and others on alleged research. It is a kindness to name none of them.

As the water content of the lens rises, so does its refractive power, thus shortening the focusing distance within the eye. Resultant loss of distance vision is compensated for by improved reading vision. As it would not be human to miss the chance of turning a frailty into an attribute, this spurious improvement is called the second sight by grandparents as they triumphantly discard their reading glasses. Unfortunately this transient second sight does not give way to a third sight until the offending lens is removed.

The final effect of cataract is to diminish central vision for near and distance. The field of vision generally suffers later. Rarely the lens may become swollen like a ripe plum, and indeed may burst within the eye, releasing toxic material into the anterior chamber, where it may inflame the iris and cause secondary glaucoma due to blockage of the drainage angle.

Symptoms

From our small group of possible complaints, the primary symptom is visual loss. Subtle questioning might elicit exaggeration of the symptoms in bright sunlight when a constricted pupil will make the cataract seem worse.

False haloes—orange rings round lights—may be mistaken for the rainbow haloes of acute glaucoma if the name halo be taken at its face value. Occasionally an opacity neatly placed in the lens will split the vision into two, resulting in double vision in one eye.

Examination

Positive signs
Central vision will be diminished, and possibly diminished more by the pinhole disc. Obstruction to the axial rays of light by a centrally placed cataract explains this phenomenon, which is almost pathognomonic of this condition. The lens opacities will appear in silhouette against the red reflex through the dilated pupil when viewed through the ophthalmoscope at a distance 8–12 in (Fig. 56).

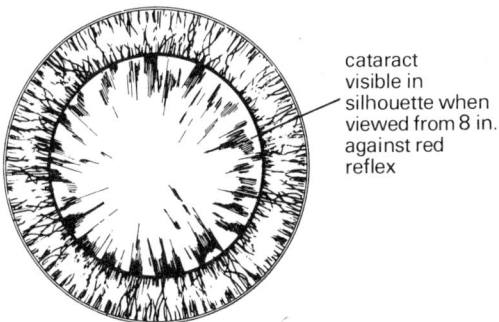

cataract visible in silhouette when viewed from 8 in. against red reflex

Fig. 56 Cataract
Discovered by the technique shown in Fig. 27

Management (adults)

The whole problem of managing cataract hinges around one simple question. Is the visual acuity bad enough to justify cataract extraction? Such an extraction, if successful, is the only sure way to eliminate this visual impediment. All other measures can only reduce the patient's awareness of this impediment.

There is a persuasive argument for avoiding cataract extraction; standard corrected vision after the cataract has been removed is very different and frequently not as pleasing as sub-standard vision with the cataract still in the eye.

As can be seen in Figure 57A, the rays of light entering the normal eye cross at the posterior surface of the normal lens. Removing a cataract and replacing the defect with a powerful spectacle lens advances the crossing point by about 2 cm. The resultant magnifying effect is well known. A policeman therefore appearing a regulation height to a normal eye will grow to disturbing proportions when presented to an eye from which a lens has been removed (aphakic) (Fig. 57B).

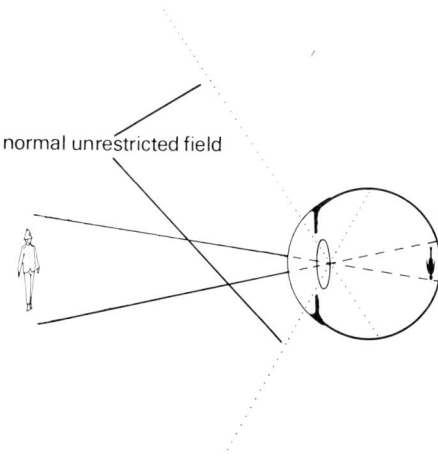

normal unrestricted field

Fig. 57A The normal image of a normal eye in a normal field

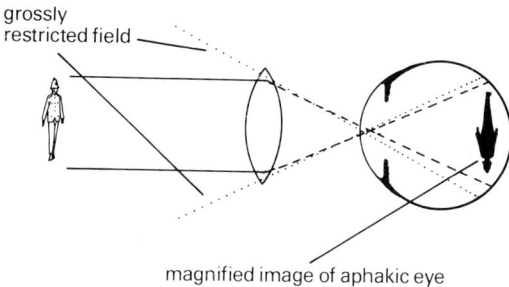

grossly restricted field

magnified image of aphakic eye

Fig. 57B The magnified image of an aphakic eye in a restricted field

The reason why a normal eye and a aphakic eye cannot be used at the same time

The visual field constricts considerably with no feathering at its peripheral edge. The result is an apparent world of magnified images that enter and leave a diminished field without warning—one moment dominant and the next moment away. It is for this reason that an aphakic eye cannot combine with a normal eye to produce binocular vision using standard glasses.

Short term

Medical
In the early stages it is sometimes possible to improve the vision by permanent dilation of the pupil with Atropine drops perhaps three times weekly. Tinting the glasses with sodium yellow may allow the light to enter but not to dazzle the eye. In addition it has the quality of making every day seem bathed in sunshine—a remarkable and priceless attribute in a British January.

Surgical
Occasionally a sector may be cut from the iris to enlarge the pupil and allow light to enter through the periphery of the lens. This is a penetrating injury, and as such may accelerate the cataract. However it might be rarely justified if the patient cannot see and the cataract, for some reason or other, cannot be removed.

Long term

Surgical
Extraction is the only effective cure. It may not be actually removing the cause, because the cause is unknown, but it is removing the results of the cause.

Preferably under general anaesthesia, an incision is made 180 degrees around the corneoscleral limbus. The lens is then lifted out either with forceps or a freezing probe. This involves dislocating the lens in its entirety from the ligaments that suspend it from the ciliary body. The younger the patient, and as far as cataracts are concerned 50 is young, the more difficult it is to dislocate the lens (Fig. 58).

In those cases the lens is deliberately ruptured and its contents evacuated, leaving behind its posterior capsule in the pupil opening. It would be necessary later to cut a hole in this capsule after the eye had recovered from the first procedure.

Whatever the procedure the corneoscleral wound is then stitched, and the patient need not be in hospital for more than four or five days. Duration of the hospital stay will vary with fashion and expense, and demand for hospital beds.

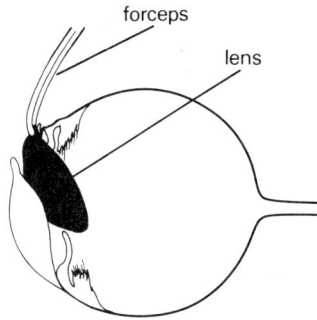

Fig. 58 Cataract extraction
There are many similarities between obstetrics and ophthalmology—not least the delivery of a reluctant object through an orifice that seems ridiculously small until the last moment

Since the operation produces a surgical iritis, the pupil will have to be dilated with Atropine drops. The inflammation may be suppressed with local corticosteroid drops.

Some eight weeks later thick glasses replacing the refractive power of the extracted lens will be prescribed.

A contact lens placed on the cornea goes some way to restoring the eye to its original optical balance. The intersection point of rays is pushed back near to where it started from, and magnification thus reduced, though not totally. However it is possible occasionally for binocular vision to be restored between a normal eye and an aphakic eye with a contact lens. There has to be the desire to succeed. There has to be the intellectual capacity to cope with the problem, and as these circumstances frequently follow a penetrating injury where goggles might have saved the eye in the first place, such intellectual capacity is not always available. If a sizeable degree of financial compensation hinges upon a failure to tolerate the contact lens, then the contact lens will usually not be tolerated.

It is also possible to fragment the cataract with an ultrasonic probe and remove the remnants by aspiration. The entry wound is considerably smaller. The stay in hospital is considerably reduced. Unfortunately, occasionally the post-operative value of the eye is also reduced by permanent damage to the corneal endothelium. In an increasing number of cases the synthetic lens may be introduced in place of the cataract either before or behind the iris. The technique naturally adds unique dangers to an operation that is already not without its own risks. However, despite its potential for complicating something simple into a catastrophe, the surgical question about these implants is gently changing from why to why not?

Management (children)

Congenital cataracts have the added dimension that macular function will develop only if allowed to. If the cataracts are dense enough to prevent this development, then they should be removed as early as is technically possible. If they are not so dense, then the same arguments about sub-standard vision apply to children just as they do to adults.

Surgical

Because the nucleus in a child's eye is not hard as it is in an adult, a congenital cataract may be aspirated up a wide bore needle. Under general anaesthesia such a needle is introduced to the pupil through the corneo-scleral limbus. As the cataract is aspirated the volume of the eye is maintained with balanced salt solution down a second needle. As far as the nucleus of a cataract is concerned, one is a child until the age of 30.

Complications

There are three major problems following cataract extraction. The first is secondary glaucoma following blockage to the angle of the anterior chamber with vitreous. This blockage does not respond to conventional surgery, because a new surgical drain would be no better than the old normal one. The problem is the vitreous—present where it ought not to be and defiant of all attempts to remove it.

The second complication is retinal detachment, which follows damage to the retinal insertion at the ora serrata.

The third complication is that the patient may not like the end result with its images too large for its visual field.

SUMMARY

A cataract can follow any insult to the eye.

Removal is justified essentially only for visual reasons, or if there is a danger that the lens, becoming soft and ripe and intumescent, may burst within the globe.

Visual justification exists if the patient cannot see with either eye, or if there is the intention to restore binocular vision in a young person with a cataract in one eye.

In children, congenital cataracts must be removed early enough to allow the development of macular function, if they are so dense that this development be threatened.

In general terms, however, if the patients are functioning happily in their own environment then they are best left alone. In that shadowy limbo where they are getting on reasonably well but not quite as well as they would like, then the pre-operative visual acuity should be such that post-operative convalescents will not think back with nostalgia to the second rate vision they had and exchanged so blithely for the unfulfilled hope of something better.

Dislocation of the lens

Spontaneous dislocation of the lens occurs in conditions where the suspensory ligament is not suspending as it ought. There is generally a galaxy of disseminated elastic and ligament malfunction throughout the body. Two classic syndromes are Marchesani's and Marfan's— bodily defects at extremes of the normal range of size. The former is short and stubby in every way, the latter tall and spidery (Fig. 59), and they both share defective joints and dislocated lenses.

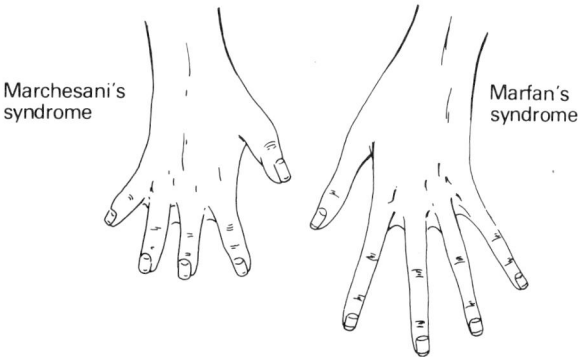

Fig. 59 The hands of Marchesani's and Marfan's syndromes
Although the slender one may appear ideally suited to the piano keyboard, the dislocated lenses prevent a clear view of the music

Pathology
If the lens merely slips, but stays in its correct plane (Fig. 60), then there may be only slight visual distortion. However, should the lens move forward then there is grave danger that it will block the drainage angle and raise the intra-ocular pressure. Movement backwards takes us into the vitreal cavity where the lens may release breakdown products of protein, toxic to the eye, which may produce vitreous haze and eventual shrinkage of the globe.

Traumatic dislocation also takes us into the old world of the travelling charlatans, who elevated the technique into an operation which they called couching the cataract. Vision was magically restored long enough for gratitude to translate itself into a more negotiable form. However at the first hint that things might be going wrong, the wanderers would exercise their talent for rapid movement, mounting a swift evasive action in search of fresh victims, whilst conveniently escaping the consequences of their most recent disasters.

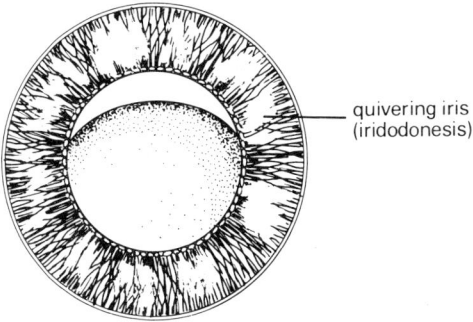
quivering iris
(iridodonesis)

Fig. 60 Lens dislocation—spontaneous or traumatic
Whatever the cause, the drainage angle and the peripheral retina must be assumed affected until proven not

Symptoms
These will generally be visual, unless secondary glaucoma produces pain.

Examination
Central vision will be diminished, but will improve with a pinhole because there is no cataract in the early stages. The iris will quiver when the pupil is examined, because the lens is not providing the support that it normally ought to. This quivering iris (iridodonesis) will clearly exist after cataract extraction for the same reason.

The finger tension will be raised in the presence of secondary glaucoma.

Management
Nothing can be done about faulty ligaments, nor can trauma be undone. The aim is then to restore vision if the vision be sufficiently affected, and to treat any secondary glaucoma that might have occurred.

13

The glaucomas

The term glaucoma can be defined as any state where the pressure of the eyeball rises above what we accept as normal. It will result from any form of blockage to the aqueous circulation at any point in its journey from the ciliary body through the pupil to the drainage angle of the anterior chamber.

If the cause be known, for example iritic adhesions at the pupil, we call it glaucoma secondary to iritis; if due to a narrow angle, we call it closed angle or acute glaucoma; if due to no recognisable cause then, with a fine sense of irony and a certain degree of effrontery, we call it *glaucoma simplex*.

By an unfortunate mischance, the term glaucoma derives from the Greek word for cataract. An eye is described as glaucous when advancing cataract gives the lens that greenish tinge allegedly associated with poor vision. In more rugged times when many eyes ended up blind and green from as many causes, the term glaucoma was applied to all of them. However, advancing knowledge has now renamed most of these according to their special pathology, but not always as helpfully as we might wish for. Because glaucoma which does not turn the eye green has retained the term glaucoma, while the original condition which actually did is now called cataract. Alas!

ACUTE GLAUCOMA (Closed angle)

The popular misconception of acute glaucoma is that it is chronic glaucoma with a degree of urgency and haloes. Unfortunately this is not the case. There is no connection in any way between the two conditions, unless someone is unfortunate enough to have both.

Acute glaucoma is not so much a disease as a shape. It occurs in the long sighted eye, with an anterior chamber too shallow for safe dilatation of the pupil. The advance of middle age exaggerates this shallowness by a forward movement of the iris lens diaphragm.

Extreme long sight has two further associates—thick glasses that obscure distant objects to all but those for whom they were prescribed, and not infrequently a convergent squint dating from childhood.

However dilatation of the pupil is not the whole story. Active contraction of the sympathetic innervated radial dilating fibres drags the iris back against the lens. Aqueous, failing to pass the pupil, pushes the peripheral iris against the angle of the anterior chamber, with sudden obstruction to the outflow.

This coup de grâce does not come out of the blue. Rather does it come out of a collection of colours known as haloes. Transient attacks of acute glaucoma raise the pressure of the eyeball and force the fluid into the cornea. Not unnaturally pain in the adjacent forehead follows the first, while blurred vision follows the second. Haloes also follow the second because the corneal oedema breaks the light into the colours of the spectrum, producing a rainbow ring—round because the cornea is round.

The anticipation of likely victims, and the prevention of such tragic attacks, is the third major aim of the ophthalmic examination. The condition is so easy to treat before it has happened that to leave it to happen borders on negligence.

We should therefore be on our guard when faced with the history of haloes. We should ask if they really mean rainbow rings, because early cataract can also ring lights with orange-red haloes, from which however some of the colours of the rainbow are missing. Thick glasses and a childhood squint should make one even more cautious, whilst the eclipse test, part of the basic ophthalmic ritual, should distinguish the shallow anterior chamber from the deep.

There was once a cinema in Edinburgh that tried to provide diversion for neglected wives to take their minds off absent husbands. They specialised in vampires, mummies and haunted castles, a perfect setting to tempt shallow fronted eyes into disaster—razor-toothed phantoms stepping from coffins and edgy long sighted squinting middle-aged housewives stumbling from the picture house in a dazzle of rainbows.

This would never have happened if someone had carried out an eclipse test and acted upon the findings.

Because dilation of the pupil alone is not the whole explanation, then constriction of the pupil alone is not the whole answer. This condition must be treated surgically. A small hole is cut in the peripheral iris (peripheral iridectomy) to allow aqueous to pass freely from its source in the ciliary body to the angle of drainage, bypassing any possible sympathetic pupil block, and eliminating haloes and all their sinister implications.

Sadly very few people with shallow fronted eyes escape a full blown attack of acute glaucoma. Indeed most of them present in the grip of one with a hazy cornea, a fixed dilated pupil and some distress. Whether the warnings were just ignored, or not marked enough to merit attention, is hard to discover because in the midst of the drama other more urgent issues come to mind. But this is in line with other ophthalmic problems. There is no shortage of complaints about things that do not matter and frequent silence about things that do.

As one happy element in the midst of these dark hazards, the misfortune rarely strikes both eyes at the same time. This may be helpful in the diagnosis, for should any doubt exist, the fellow eye, which should be examined anyway, may by its shallow anterior chamber give a clue to the behaviour of the first.

The condition is an ocular emergency, and delay can result in blindness, followed by an attack in the second eye.

The pressure must be reduced immediately. Acetazolamide, if necessary by intravenous injection (500 mg), will cut down the aqueous flow from the ciliary body. Pilocarpine drops (2 per cent) poured in intensively may constrict the pupil sufficiently to open the drainage angle. The same drops in a rather smaller dosage (four times a day), though no guarantee, may tip the balance against a similar attack in the fellow eye (Figs 61, 62 & 63).

Surgical treatment will be necessary. As it is likely that the drainage angle will have been damaged by a prolonged attack of glaucoma, then a permanent fistula cut into the sclera will allow aqueous drainage into the subconjunctival space. Clearly this is not a procedure to carry out lightly; firstly, it does not always work; secondly, it sometimes works too well; and thirdly, however it works, its disturbance of the aqueous dynamics may be enough to cause cataract.

Until the first eye has recovered from surgery, a low dosage of Pilocarpine drops may temporarily protect the second eye until a peripheral iridectomy makes this protection complete.

CHRONIC GLAUCOMA

Chronic glaucoma is a most sinister and tragic cause of blindness— sinister because it is usually symptomless until gross field loss can no longer be ignored, and tragic because it could have been arrested in the first place. If patients have heard at all about glaucoma, it will be the acute painful variety. Otherwise, they ascribe any visual loss to cataract, which they have all heard about and which they all usually get wrong too.

Chronic glaucoma may be defined as any rise of intra-ocular pressure above what we call normal and for which no cause can be found. *In normal circumstances there is a happy balance between the pressure of blood supplying the optic nerve head and the pressure of the eyeball itself.*

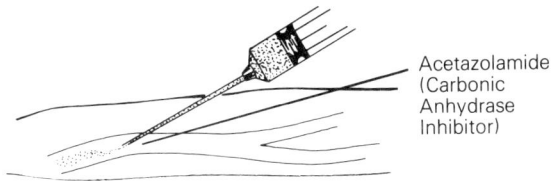

Acetazolamide (Carbonic Anhydrase Inhibitor)

Fig. 61

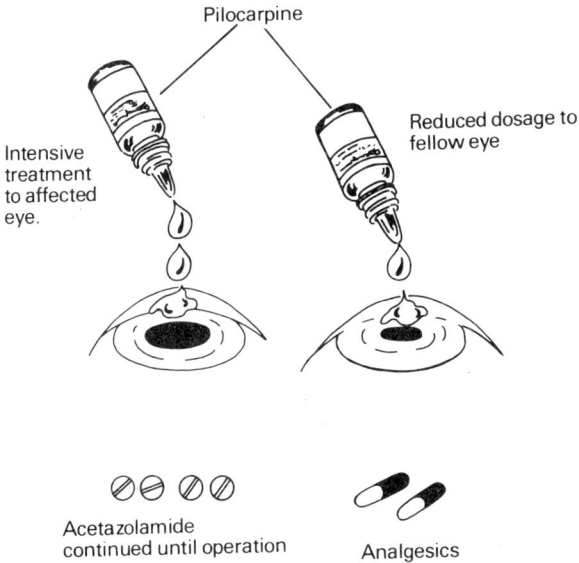

Pilocarpine

Intensive treatment to affected eye.

Reduced dosage to fellow eye

Acetazolamide continued until operation

Analgesics

Fig. 62

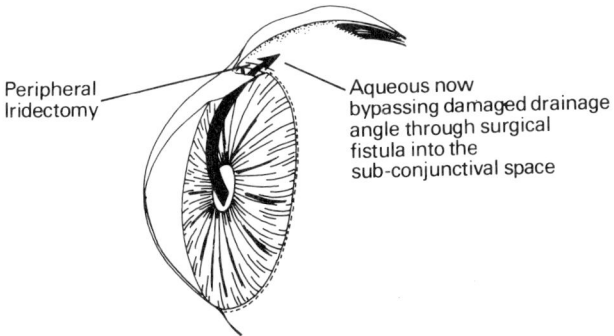

Peripheral Iridectomy

Aqueous now bypassing damaged drainage angle through surgical fistula into the sub-conjunctival space

Fig. 63

Figs 61, 62, 63 The treatment of acute glaucoma
If neglected this emergency leads to the needless loss of one eye and possibly its fellow if misdiagnosed. The anterior chamber is shallow in both (Eclipse test) although possibly visible only in one

However, in glaucoma this balance is upset, and a battle develops in its place between the pressure of blood trying to get into the optic nerve head and the intra-ocular pressure now trying to stop it. If the intra-ocular pressure wins, then the capillary closure begins to starve, in the first instance, those nerve fibres that provide vision in arcs above and below the fixation point.

Appropriate field defects now develop, which because of their position are allowed to continue to develop unnoticed. The defects are almost always well clear of the central visual line, and discovery is further delayed because the visual field is served by two eyes. However to monocular testing, any defects would be detectable first of all on the nasal side. There are very few symptoms until it is too late, and it is only by good fortune that both eyes are not carried off at the same time.

Although our classic aim is to dispel pain, these classic signs might never be allowed to develop were pain a feature of chronic glaucoma.

In the early stages of the condition, not only may there be no symptoms, there may be no signs either. The fields, were we to examine them, would be full, the discs would be healthy. Even a spot assessment of the intra-ocular pressure would be within what we call normal limits. This last tends to fluctuate throughout the day, and it is the swing of intra-ocular pressure, rising above normal occasionally, that eventually leads into a pathological state where the pressure is permanently raised.

At this point signs begin to develop. The central cup, normally occupying a quarter of the optic disc, begins to enlarge vertically (Fig. 64). And the enlargement is reflected in corresponding gaps in the visual field.

These classic gaps form in patches along a line circling from the blind spot widely around the macula. The patches coalesce quietly and creep inwards and outwards, whilst the patient reads the smallest print, happily unaware of impending doom. A two yearly, competent examination of the eyes as well as of their refractive errors, before there is any hint that all is not well, will avert this doom while it is still impending.

Treatment

Treatment aims to bring the intra-ocular pressure down to a level where the field defects become static. To eliminate the actual cause is still a despairing wish. To arrest it, however, is a reasonable one, and this is achieved in two basic ways:

1. Aqueous outflow is increased.
2. Aqueous inflow is decreased.

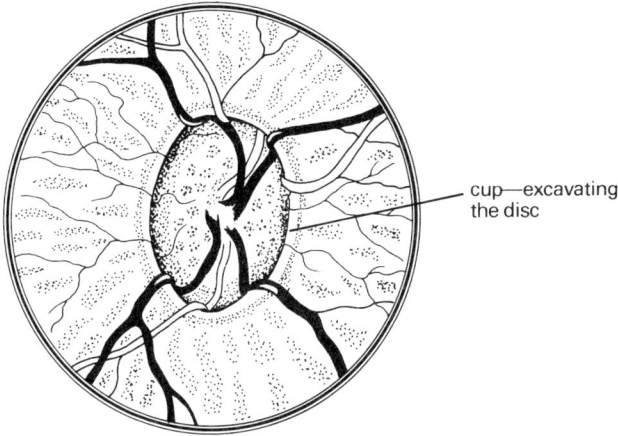

cup—excavating
the disc

Fig. 64 Glaucoma
A grossly cupped optic disc—the tragic result of not having the eyes examined until after something goes wrong—or of incompetent examination before something has gone wrong—and occasionally after. A safe eye is one that does not harbour an undiagnosed glaucoma

Pilocarpine
This parasympathomimetic agent, in some as yet unclarified way, encourages the outflow of aqueous when it has begun to falter. A hundred years of research have told us no more than the fact that it happens. As the same hundred years have been equally uninformative about the normal drainage of aqueous from the eye, it is not surprising that we have not yet penetrated the mysteries of how the effective drugs work.

The pupil constriction so acceptable in acute closed angle glaucoma becomes an unwanted side effect in the open angle variety. It darkens the vision; it drags on the muscle of accommodation; it makes the eye short sighted: it also makes a patient with such symptoms wonder why the glaucoma clinic staff are so delighted with their management of a condition that had no symptoms before treatment was started.

Adrenaline
If Pilocarpine reduces the intra-ocular pressure by some autonomic action, so paradoxically does Adrenaline, enhancing the outflow and eventually reducing the inflow. Exactly how it achieves this is perhaps a sterile question, for both effects are minimal.

The action of adrenaline is potentiated when the sympathetic system is paralysed. Guanethedine, although discredited in the treatment of hypertension because of erratic absorption, can produce such a paralysis when applied locally. A composite preparation containing Adrenaline and Guanethedine is available but it seems more prone to inflame the outside of the eye than to reduce the pressure within it.

Timolol maleate

To complete this autonomic circle of paradox, the beta adrenergic receptor blocking agents also reduce the intra-ocular pressure, mainly by decreasing the inflow of aqueous. These drugs and the eye did not start off happily together. The systemic drug Practolol, effective against hypertension, was more effective still against mucous membranes. Its analogue Timolol has not been implicated in any such disasters.

Unlike Pilocarpine and Adrenaline it neither constricts nor dilates the pupil. However systemic absorption may slow the heart rate dangerously in the presence of congestive cardiac failure, and any tendency to bronchial spasm may extend into a frank attack of asthma. And, although patients may see again through a normal pupil, they may well not appreciate the visual improvement if they now cannot breathe. Fortunately the incidence is not high.

Acetazolamide

This drug, now discarded as a diuretic, has regained a place in medicine by its very significant reduction in aqueous production. Although complicated from time to time by potassium loss or metabolic acidosis, it may have a place in the treatment of those whose fingers are too stiff to manipulate bottles or whose memories are too wayward to remember. Nausea and finger tip paraesthesiae may make a change of treatment necessary, and it should not be forgotten that Acetazolamide was not used as the original diuretic for nothing.

Surgery

By all these measures a progression of chronic field loss is halted. Regular examination is required to ensure that the arrested field loss does not break out again from its medical confines. Should it do so, then the decision gradually and reluctantly edges towards surgery.

Glaucoma operations aim to drain off aqueous through a permanent fistula into the sub-conjunctival space. The body does not approve of such unnatural channels and may close them off with fibrous tissue, especially in the younger patients.

Fortunately the older eyes, where they are most often required, do not close off the drain so successfully. This cannot, however, be taken for granted. Even if successful, these operations do, however, upset aqueous dynamics, and may give rise to cataract formation over the years.

Glaucoma is one of these impossible conditions where doctor and patient are frequently at loggerheads. To start with, patients come for a new lens in their old frames and end up with Pilocarpine. We tell them they are doing well, and they tell us they cannot see.

If they default with the Pilocarpine and the central visual acuity improves we cut short their pleasure with a lecture on doing what they are told.

Acetazolamide at this point may make them feel unwell enough to deflect attention from their eyes to nausea, tingling fingers and occasional incontinence.

And when with stoical embarrassment they have become resigned to all these inconveniences we tell them they need surgery, which may result in cataract even if successful. Indeed it may produce cataract anyway when not successful, though by this time the human capacity for making the best of a bad job will brace their resolve for further intervention, the reason for which they had long ceased to question.

Timolol, however, hopefully is pointing the way out of these thickets. Still a parvenue of suspect pedigree, it may not be welcomed in circles where the shortcomings of Pilocarpine have been balanced by the experience of a century. However there is always a niche for the successful, despite its relations, and caution should add time to verify first impressions.

Timolol is now seriously challenging the role of Pilocarpine, and if this challenge be successful, the old order will give way to a new order, when patients will not only retain their vision but they will continue to see at the same time.

SECONDARY GLAUCOMA

When the intra-ocular pressure rises in response to any other recognisable agency we use the term secondary glaucoma. Strictly speaking all glaucomas are secondary to something. It is just that in chronic simple glaucoma we do not yet know to what. Because closed angle glaucoma is always due to the same thing, it has been granted a title in its own right.

Congenital malfunction of the draining angle, traumatic scarring of the draining angle, diabetic new vessel formation in the draining angle, iritic debris anywhere, and many other affronts from the inventory of causes can block aqueous flow either within the eye at the pupil or on its way out (Fig. 65).

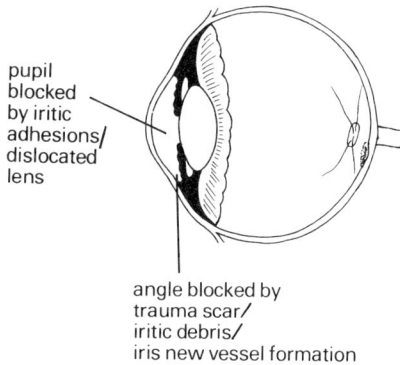

pupil
blocked
by iritic
adhesions/
dislocated
lens

angle blocked by
trauma scar/
iritic debris/
iris new vessel formation

Fig. 65 Secondary glaucoma
The circulation of aqueous may be obstructed at many points by many
conditions. The condition may be obvious; the aqueous obstruction may not. Once
again the patient does not recognise that the field is going until it is gone

When the drama of the primary condition has settled, any
secondary glaucoma may destroy the visual field as silently as does its
famous namesake.

To foresee and forestall this wanton destruction we must always
remember the continuing marvel of aqueous production and aqueous
drainage, and that while other parts of the eye will offer a diagnostic
plethora of symptoms and signs, the aqueous flow will suffer in silence
until the effects of its suffering will be discovered when it is already
too late. To be alert to such a possibility is the first step to diagnosis.

Management has two basic elements. Because the pressure is high it
must be brought down, usually with Acetazolamide, to a level where
the field loss is arrested. The pupillary constriction of Pilocarpine is
not the safest line of action, especially in the presence of iritis, where
anything but would be indicated. Pilocarpine is therefore not
recommended until its safety be established. The second element is to
deal with the exciting cause.

Reversible conditions like acute iritis, which silt up the drainage
angle with inflammatory debris, must be reversed, usually with
medical measures. A surgical peripheral iridectomy can bypass the
pupillary adhesions of chronic iritis. Traumatic scarring of the
drainage meshwork might be handled just like chronic glaucoma. The
variations of management depend on what is the least damaging
alternative to leaving the primary condition untreated, remembering
that not only must the retina be protected, it must also continue to be
accessible to light through a transparent cornea, lens and vitreous.

14

Nystagmus

Nystagmus may be defined as an involuntary purposeless repetitive oscillation of one or both eyes in any direction at any speed and at any frequency. Although lengthy, this definition at least has the advantage of being beyond discussion. Its precise significance, however, unfortunately is not.

Nystagmus occurs when some lesion produces a defect in the normal mechanisms that initiate or direct ocular movements. The third, fourth and sixth cranial nerves, linked to each other and to their fellows across the brain stem by the medial longitudinal bundles, control the six muscles which move each eye, and several factors control the nerves (Fig. 66).

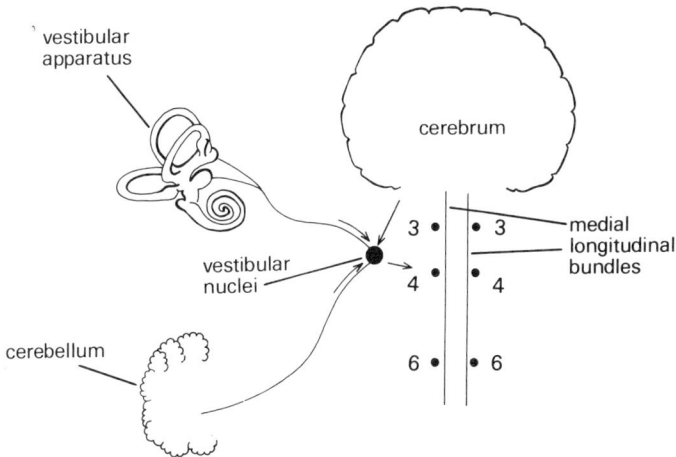

Fig. 66 Factors controlling normal eye movements

The peripheral retina flits and hovers through the available images in the field of vision before offering its selection to the macular central vision. After interpretation in the occipital cortex these flat pictures from each eye are then fused into stereoscopic binocular vision. Impulses from the cerebral cortex may over-ride subcortical muscle control, and might move the eyes from one field towards a totally new one of it own choosing. However several other mechanisms in their turn influence the voluntary cortex.

The otoliths give the eye information about the position of the head in space.

The semi-circular canals supply information about movement of the head in space.

The cerebellum via the vestibular nuclei imposes a refined restraint on the natural coarseness of eye movements, as indeed it does on any other muscular activity—a mysterious mechanism like so many other human faculties appreciated only when it has ceased to function properly.

It must now be clear that the cause of nystagmus may either lie in the eye or in the head. And since most controlling elements are found within the head, then most causative lesions must be there also, although they are not always found.

TYPES OF NYSTAGMUS

Ocular

A child born with some impairment of fixation, whether it be due to a corneal opacity, congenital cataract or albinism, has no mechanism for holding the eyes still in any position of gaze. The eyes therefore develop a pendular searching movement for a point of repose that for ever eludes them. The movements are of equal speed and amplitude in all directions.

Latent nystagmus

As the name implies, the condition is present only when a dominant eye is obscured—for example during the cover test. It is superfluous to admit that the cause is generally unknown.

Intra-cranial nystagmus

The movements here are not of equal speed. There is a fast component, a slow component, and the eyes may jerk in as many directions as the eyes can move.

Analysing these various components, experts in neurology can occasionally locate what part of the brain is at fault. The rest of us should be content with something less. Intra-cranial nystagmus naturally divides into those of long standing and those of recent origin.

Long standing nystagmus

There is usually someone on hand to confirm the reputation for wandering eyes, and in any case the patient's survival must show that, although the exact position of the disease is unknown, its effect on life expectancy is not.

Nystagmus of recent onset
Generally it is one of an abundance of signs that make the observation of nystagmus merely an interesting addition to the list. But there is, however, one condition where nystagmus is the only presenting member of the list.

In children, a posterior fossa tumour, bereft of other symptoms in its early stages, may cause the eyes to jerk quickly to one side and slowly to the other. It must be distinguished from other causes of nystagmus common in the same age group—ocular nystagmus, where the eyes do not jerk, and latent nystagmus, not present with both eyes open.

The parental observation of recent onset should eliminate any tragic misdiagnosis, though the certainly malignant pathology would temper any pleasure that might come from being correct.

End point nystagmus
In states of general fatigue and languor, people may find it difficult to maintain their chosen ocular position in extremes of lateral gaze. The eyes keep drifting back to the centre, and the person corrects this drift with a fast movement back to the original lateral position (Fig. 67). This fast movement is not purposeless.

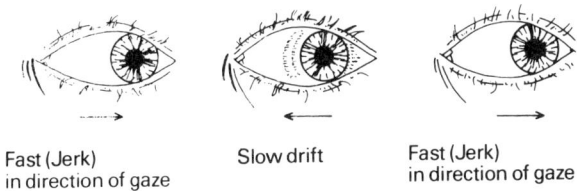

Fast (Jerk)   Slow drift   Fast (Jerk)
in direction of gaze   in direction of gaze

Fig. 67 End point nystagmus

It is important to note that this end point drift occurs only in lateral gaze, never in the straightforward position, and the direction of the fast movement changes from one side to the other. The uninhibited consumption of intoxicating fluids may produce the same condition.

Occurring in one eye only, this may be the first sign of a frank sixth nerve palsy.

Spasmus nutans
Very occasionally a six-month-old baby embarks on the strange course

of apparently pointless head nodding, while jerking the eyes around in an asymmetric and equally pointless way. Since so much else of one's behaviour at six months may appear pointless, it is wiser to take such a view of the spasmus nutans. The habit is of no consequence, and an affected child will happily return to normality within a few months before hospital investigation has put this likelihood at risk.

15

Eyes that squint

The eyes normally move together in parallel to extend that range of vision which is already made available by the swivelling and nodding action of the head upon the neck.

They can also move against each other out of parallel when they converge to focus on a near object—a reflex but recently acquired in the process of evolution, and often the first to vanish when the shocks of existence become too much to bear.

Six muscles supplied by three nerves are responsible for the movements of each eye. In reverse order their action is as follows:

The sixth nerve to the lateral rectus moves the eye outwards.

The fourth nerve to the superior oblique turns the eye downwards when it is in the converged position for reading.

The third nerve supplies all other movements. In addition it raises the upper lid and forms the outflow part of the pupil reflexes carrying the impulses for constriction.

The entire arrangement is designed to point both eyes at the same object at the same time to achieve perception in depth. This faculty is called *binocular vision*. That it works is clear, but how it works is perhaps not so clear. None the less its influence can be neatly demonstrated by someone trying to catch a bouncing rugby ball with both eyes open, then with one closed (Fig. 68).

Squinting eyes fall naturally into two groups:

1. Those without binocular vision.
2. Those with binocular vision.

The distinction is critical. In the first group, because the eyes cannot work together they work separately. But because they are pointing in different directions they therefore cannot work at the same time. The result is the alternating use of either eye, or the habitual use of one eye, whilst the other lapses into lazy amblyopia.

The second group do work together, because the brain has learned to interpret their simultaneous flow of similar images. Separation of these eyes, classically by a paralysed muscle, will produce a

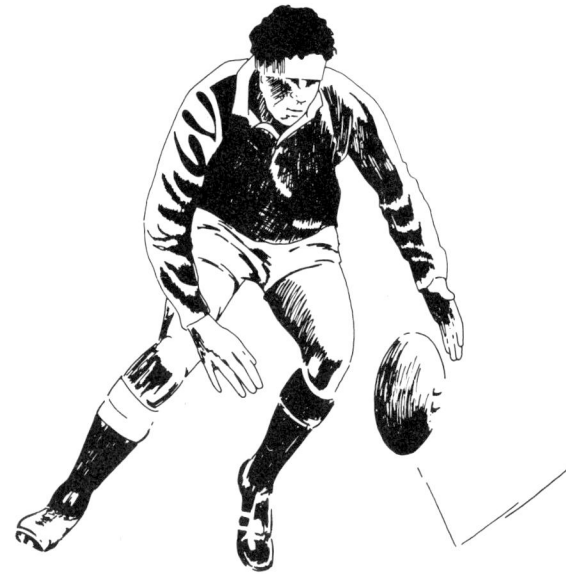

Fig. 68 Binocular vision
To catch a bouncing rugby ball is one of its supreme tests. If binocular vision is present the classic childhood squint is not; its presence can be proved

simultaneous flow of wholly dissimilar images. Each eye will continue to see, but not the same thing, and the result is a bitter complaint of double vision.

EYES WITHOUT BINOCULAR VISION

Most squinting eyes will squint because there is no binocular vision to hold them together. However other factors occasionally interfere. Simple light deprivation by ptosis or a congenital cataract will prevent the development of macular function. Because the mechanisms of focus and convergence are closely linked, the overuse of the first when long sighted eyes attempt to make out near detail will lead to excessive use of the second, and the eyes will converge beyond the range of the binocular lock.

While central vision is still developing, it can just as easily stop developing. Rather than tolerate the confusion of double images, the brain will suppress the desire for both eyes to work at once. If the eyes are equal the suppression will alternate from one to the other. If the eyes are unequal the child will favour the one with the lesser spectacle error. The longer the suppression continues the more difficult will it be to reverse, and by the age of five reversal is usually impossible and the child will be committed to the use of one eye at a time.

It is for this reason that squint must be discovered early. The child will not grow out of a squint. The price of neglect is the macular function of one eye.

At the other end of the scale there is a lower age limit below which examination will only confirm to little patients what they already knew, that hospitals are not to be tolerated. By the age of one year, children are generally prepared to co-operate for a while, and not to concentrate their entire minds on escape.

Not all squints are in fact squints. A common occurrence is an apparent squint produced by facial asymmetry. Every face has unequal sides. Some are just more unequal than other. Exaggerated skin folds from the upper lid to the nose (epicanthus), a racial characteristic normally in South-east Asian peoples but not in others, can give the impression of abnormally convergent eyes (Fig. 69).

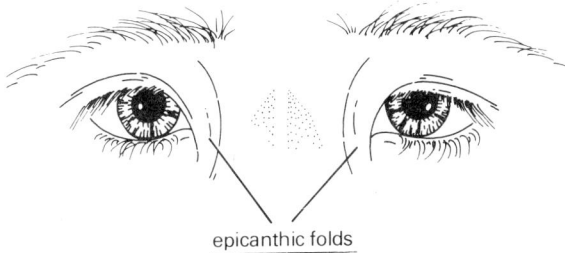

epicanthic folds

Fig. 69 Epicanthic folds
What appears to be a squint is not always a squint

That these folds will recede spontaneously has not prevented impatient surgeons from attempting to hasten their recession with the knife. And children, tormented at school with the nickname of 'Slit Eyes', have been known tearfully to report the new sobriquet of 'Scarface'.

Because the whole point of treatment is to improve and maintain macular fixation, the second point in examination is therefore to see if macular fixation is in fact present in both eyes.

Most parents are prepared for the cosmetic defect, but the threat to central vision can test their resilience, as indeed our explanation may test their comprehension. They may not recover sufficiently from either to co-operate in treatment.

The cover test
There is a widespread notion that a squint must settle in one eye or the other. Like so many other popular beliefs, this is just not true.

Squinting eyes deviate from each other at a fixed angle. When one eye looks straight ahead the other does not, and the angle between them is the angle of the squint. If the second eye can now be persuaded to look straight ahead, the first will now no longer, and the angle between them remains the same unchanged angle of the squint.

Habitual fixation with one eye does not alter this fact. It merely tells us that the macular function on that side is too good ever to let the macular function on the other side take over by itself. Nevertheless the angle of the squint still remains a fixed angle between both eyes.

The cover test is simply a manoeuvre to demonstrate this angle (Fig. 70). Because it is a test of fixation, we must make sure that the child is in fact looking at an object of our choice lest we come to a false conclusion when he was looking at an object of his own choice. Fixing objects vary. A torch is just another light, but a stick decorated with little pictures, like policemen, teddy bears and colourful birds, can be more persuasive. These pictures should have enough detail to stimulate near focus, when an actual squint may become quite obvious. Indeed it may be the only time it becomes obvious except when the struggle to focus against Atropine paralysis exaggerates the squinting tendency.

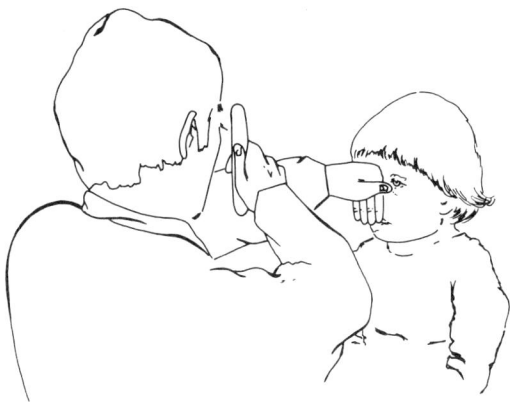

Fig. 70 The Cover test
How to elicit the details of Fig. 71 in a child who has no binocular vision

Fixation on the stick can be made quite certain when a slight side to side waggle of the stick will excite corresponding side to side movements in the child's eyes. By placing a hand before first one eye then the other, we can demonstrate this horse rein action of both eyes as they swing at their fixed angle between alternating fixation on the stick. The covered eye will move towards a squinting position, whilst the uncovered eye will move into the straight ahead position (Fig. 71).

The entire movement will be reversed but equal when the other eye is covered.

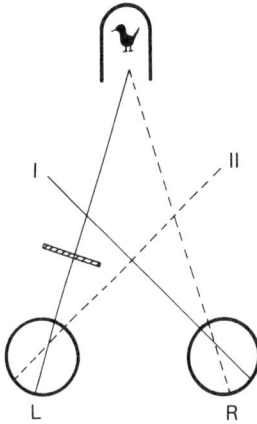

Position I
L eye fixing
R eye convergent at a particular angle.
Position II
L eye covered
R eye now moved out to fix
L eye follows it in like the reins of a horse. *The angle of squint remains unchanged.*

Fig. 71 What the Cover test reveals
        Most often unhappily, only to those who do it often

If there is no squint there will be no movement.

The eye movements tested separately will be full and equal with each other. The eyes are just set at the wrong angle. The angle does not vary. There is no muscle paralysis. The child cannot complain of double vision.

A test for binocular vision

If a child thought to squint has demonstrable binocular vision, then the chances are he has no squint. The presence of three-dimensional vision can be proved when flat polarised images spring to life when viewed through polarised spectacles. There is such a test—the 'Stereoscopic Fly' whose cartoon characters should compete successfully for the attention of the average two-year-old. At this point an equivocal cover test ceases to matter.

Management

The pupils must be dilated to allow an objective measurement of spectacle error, for many children are either unwilling or unable to recognise a subjective improvement in a spectacle frame. Mydriasis also allows us to eliminate diseases of the retina, which just occasionally could be a retinoblastoma.

Once a squint has been demonstrated then the child is handed over to the orthoptists who are well practised in wheedling information out of truculent three year olds. If the central vision of one eye be reduced even with appropriate glasses then they will set out on a course of patching. This involves occlusion of the good eye during the waking hours for something like a month at a time, to force the poorer eye to drive its functional pathway through to the brain.

Although these explanations may be conducted amidst smiling goodwill, it is the mother who has to deal with all the tantrums and defiance during the period of occlusion. It is vital that it be carried out ruthlessly by a combination of cajolery and resistance to tearful promises of good behaviour tomorrow, if only the patch can come off today.

The aim of treatment is to establish equal macular vision. Once the child is capable of fixing alternately with either eye, the visual pathways have been established. Should the central vision of one eye later decline because the other is preferred, it can always be restored should it ever be needed as the only eye. If, however, the macula has never established a free passage for impulses to the brain then all the expensive intercessions so readily available to anxious parents will not make it do so.

Surgery

Surgery, generally for cosmetic reasons, is usually the last step in the line of treatment. In some countries where such a service is not readily available or welcomed, an imposing squint may be considered a token of military genius, or at least a delivery system for evil rays. Such prized qualities, often leading to tribal leadership, will not be lightly exchanged for a comely appearance.

When surgery is considered, however, the ideal time is just before a child goes to school, when his fellows' facility for wounding nicknames will be frustrated. Since this child does not have binocular vision, the eyes once straightened may finally diverge, because the orbits point outwards anyway. Such divergence can of course be reversed by further surgery some years later still.

Amblyopia

To complete our list of popular misconceptions, it is commonly believed that a lazy eye (amblyopic) must be a squinting eye. Now while most squinting eyes may become lazy, not all lazy eyes squint. They may be straight, but deprived of macular stimulation by anything that interferes with the fixing mechanism—from ptosis through congenital cataract to glasses unworn when glasses should be worn.

A gross difference in refraction such as prevents binocular vision in people who try to match an aphakic eye with a normal eye, has the same effect as eyes that have just been born that way. Correction of these extreme spectacle errors at an early age is necessary to educate the brain to accept this discrepancy. If correction has been neglected or rejected, then we have up to the time of the early teens to force the lazy eye into action when patching the other will make it work on its own.

EYES WITH BINOCULAR VISION

After full binocular vision has formed, anything that makes one visual axis deviate from its fellow will result in two distinct images which separate in proportion to the deviation. There are three conditions which result in this, and in all of them the symptoms will vanish when one eye is covered.

Latent squint

In nobody are the eyes absolutely straight. There is always a slight hidden deviation, normally overcome by a powerful binocular lock. These deviations become significant only when the eyes would prefer to separate rather further from each other than the brain can tolerate.

Symptoms of transient double vision and difficulty in depth perception now depend on how quickly such people pull their eyes together, and on how much their lives revolve around a fine binocular capacity. If another stress be added, then the binocular lock may just break apart. A classic example of this came to light during the war when certain pilots found it impossible to judge their returning height from the runway—an understandable lapse of judgement if the Luftwaffe were not far behind. A modification of the cover test can unmask this condition.

The cover-uncover test

This test of binocularity must therefore end with both eyes uncovered. Otherwise the elements of fixation, the side to side waggle and the occluding hand are very much as before.

This time we must carefully watch the movement of the hidden eye when the covering hand is removed. It will be seen to swing from its wrong direction back into the straight position. There is no horse rein action. The fellow eye remains motionless. Binocular vision has come into play again. The whole process can be repeated, this time using the other eye (Figs 72 & 73).

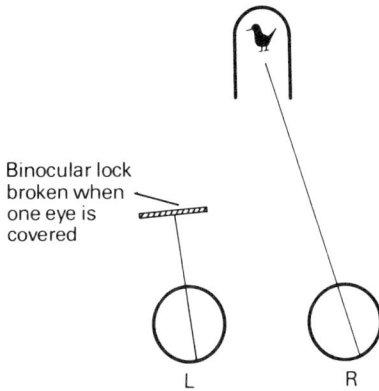

Binocular lock
broken when
one eye is
covered

L   R

Left eye drifting outwards.
Its mechanical position taking precedence in
the absence of binocular instructions

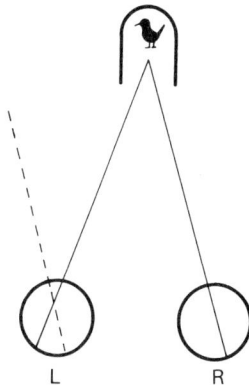

L   R

Cover now removed.
Left eye has now swung back to join its static fellow.
Binocular instructions now taking precedence
over mechanical position

Figs 72, 73 The Cover-uncover test
The recognition of eyes whose binocular desire and actual position are at
odds with each other

The distance of the correcting movement tells us the extent of the condition. The speed with which the eye moves over this distance will determine the brain's eagerness to overcome the mechanical separation.

The absence of a muscle palsy will tell us that the condition is benign.

If accurate lens prescription fails to relieve the symptoms, orthoptic exercises can sometimes make them seem better, though leaving the deviation just as it was before. The improvement, if any, is purely subjective. If there is no improvement then the deviation itself may be reduced by altering the position of the eyes. Not infrequently such a threat makes the previously scorned orthoptic exercises appear just the treatment the patient had in mind.

Convergence weakness

Young people, especially when faced with some debilitating experience like studying on a sunny summer evening or imminent exposure at an examination, may develop double vision for near objects. They lose their ability to converge the eyes, find grave difficulty with reading and produce an irrefutable reason for not staying in to study.

There is no muscle palsy. The eyes can look both left and right but cannot converge to read. The complaint can be verified by the development of double images of the fixation stick before it has come within the normal reading distance.

If the general health is good and normal muscle movements confirmed, then exercises may help to bring the convergence point nearer to the nose. As the evenings shorten in the winter so does the convergence distance. Adults with no particular confrontation to avoid can suffer the same condition and will respond just as well to the same treatment. In both situations any necessary spectacles should be prescribed.

Muscular paralysis

Any disease from the brain stem to the orbit may cause a muscle to malfunction. The commonest is head injury, which can produce anything from simple bruising to total destruction of the brain.

Intra-cranial lesions, such as an aneurysm or a brain tumour, are more common in the younger age groups, while diabetes, hypertension and arteriosclerosis are associated with the older age groups.

Fluctuating double vision, worsening towards the end of the day, is almost diagnostic of myasthenia gravis, whilst a muscle palsy as part of an unconnected catalogue of signs must raise the spectre of multiple sclerosis.

Thiamine deficiency can have an equally widespread influence, dislocating the mind and the nervous control of the muscles from the eyes to the legs—the Wernicke-Korsakoff syndrome. With today's intake of alcohol now rivalling that of the Regency period, there is no shortage of alcoholics who might starve themselves into a state of double vision, ataxia and a skein of confusion and fabrication. The condition can be relieved by intra-muscular injections of Thiamine; it can be fatal without them.

Whatever the underlying cause, a paralysed muscle in a conscious patient with developed binocular vision must produce double vision; this double vision increases when the paralysed muscle is put under stress.

Testing the eye movements is therefore mandatory. A separate examination of each eye should precede the test with both eyes open—not as an ophthalmic examination, but as part of the general cranial nerve examination which can and should be briefly completed in these circumstances.

If the double vision be genuine, and frequently it is not, then investigation should be limited to urinalysis for sugar, blood pressure, a full blood count, and possibly radiographs of the skull.

In younger people double vision must always be taken seriously, and even in the absence of headaches, serious intra-cranial disease must be assumed until disproved. However since such investigations may leave the patient worse off than he was when he started, they should not be undertaken lightly.

SUMMARY

In all people there is a tendency for the eyes to drift apart when one or both are covered.

In most people this latent tendency is kept latent by the binocular lock.

In some people a pronounced tendency may, with added stress, break the binocular lock.

In all people with developed binocular vision a paralysed extra-ocular muscle will also break the binocular lock.

In most children who squint, there is no binocular lock.

16

Retinal detachment

A retinal detachment is not really a detachment at all, but a separation of two distinct retinal layers. However the term detachment, lingering from the pioneering days of ophthalmology, has lingered too long to tolerate substitution. The neuro-retina and the pigment retina normally give up their independent existence to fuse into a composite epithelium which secretes aqueous from the deep surface of the ciliary body before ending its journey forwards as the deep layer of the iris (Fig. 74).

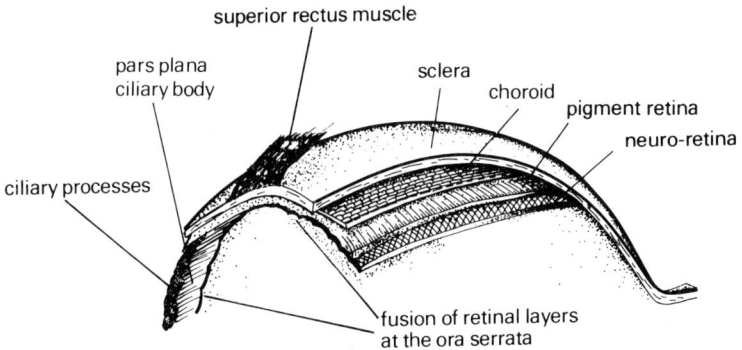

Fig. 74 The ocular layers
The two retinal layers fuse at the ora serrata, posterior to which separation of one retina from the other is called a retinal detachment. The rectus insertions are the scleral landmark of the ora serrata

The transformation from two layers to one layer takes place in a scalloped line, more remembered perhaps for its quaint name of ora serrata than for its actual position. Marking the anterior limit of the functioning retina, this ora serrata lies deep to a line connecting the insertions of the four rectus muscles. Any injury perforating the globe behind this line will certainly perforate the retina as well, and as certainly cause it to detach. The two layers are adherent also at the optic nerve head, but a potential space remains between them everywhere else. When we talk of retinal detachment we mean that the potentially mobile neuro-retina has for some reason abandoned its natural position of contact with the outer pigment retina. The vitreous body, that transparent substance like waterglass, is also attached to the retina at the same two points, namely, the optic nerve head and the ora serrata. An intact vitreous permanently keeps the retina in place. However, the passing years reduce the viscosity of the vitreous, a process exaggerated by injury or extreme myopia. This is the first step along the road to separation of the two layers that we call retinal detachment.

The commonest cause of retinal detachment is a break in the retina through which passes liquid vitreous separating the neural layer from the pigment layer. Once separated this neural layer begins to starve, and if left long enough will starve to death becoming in the process so fibrotic that mechanical replacement would be impossible even if enough functioning retina remained to justify the surgical attempt.

Abnormal adhesion of the vitreous to the retina facilitates the formation of retinal breaks. Repetitive traction on this adhesion will stimulate the retina into the only response left available by its high degree of specialisation—light flashing. As the retina tears, the flashing lights stop, though rupture of a blood vessel may fill the vitreous cavity with blood and the visual field with a sudden shower of floaters—like a swarm of bees. Later on if the jelly be thin enough the two layers will separate, producing a corresponding defect in the visual field.

If sudden, this will appear dramatically. If less sudden, the mild symptoms may be ignored until the separating retina lifts the macula and brings the patient for consultation six months after the process has started, as an urgent case of visual loss.

There are four main types of retinal detachment and all of them, unless vitreous haemorrhage has obscured the view, are characterised by a grey rippling reflex in place of the normal red reflex (Fig. 75). The normally transparent retina, seen in profile along its substance, becomes opaque and obscures the underlying choroidal red glow. The retinal vessels closer to the lens seem blacker when clockwise rotation of the ophthalmoscopic disc brings them into focus. And that may be about all it brings into focus because the direct ophthalmoscope begins to falter when it reaches towards the equator and unfortunately it is beyond the equator that any significant detachment pathology is to be found.

Myopia

Myopic eyes with not enough retina to go round their larger globe, and a correspondingly thin vitreous, are much more likely to develop

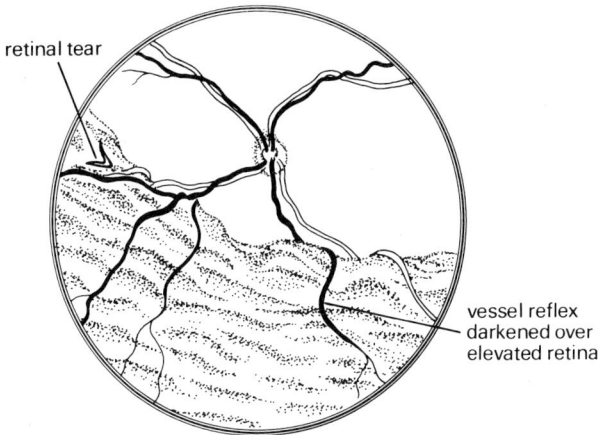

Fig. 75 Retinal detachment showing an arrowhead tear
Another breach in the treaty of background appearance. The mottled choroid visible through the neural retina, transparent when flat, is obscured by the neural retina, grey when detached

holes in the retina—a tendency exaggerated often by trivial disturbance. Myopes, not only bookish, are frequently musical as well, and it is perhaps surprising that more virtuosi do not retire from the keyboard in the midst of a savage cadenza and a shower of sparks.

After cataract extraction
Cataract removal leaves a space into which the vitreous advances, tugging on its normal attachment to the retina at the ora serrata. While more common in less happy cataract extractions, it can mar the nicest of surgical manoeuvres and indeed one's reputation, unless the possibility be clearly defined to the patient before cataract surgery is undertaken.

Trauma
A blow to the eye can rip the retina from its moorings in the extreme periphery. It should be remembered that such a blow can also dislocate the lens and produce scarring of the drainage angle with consequent secondary glaucoma.

Congenital
Maldevelopment of the retina may produce retinal cracks parallel and adjacent to the lower ora serrata. Gravity and a healthy vitreous delay the advance of this detachment, which the patient may fail to notice until the macula succumbs.

Surgery

The aim of surgery is to find the retinal break, and this can only be done satisfactorily with the indirect ophthalmoscope—it will be remembered that the view with direct ophthalmoscope fails to reach anterior to the equator. Inflammation is then induced around the break from outside the eye, the current vogue being a freezing pencil (Fig. 76). The retinal layers around the break are then held together watertight until the inflammation induces a scar, also hopefully

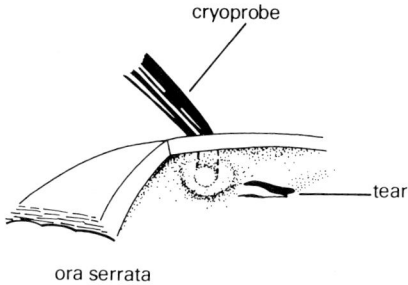

Fig. 76 Freezing all the layers of the eye around a retinal tear
The *sine qua non* of effective detachment surgery

watertight. Because of the dangers of persisting traction on the retina which may pull open the tear again, it is customary to reduce the volume of the eye by some form of scleral buckling. This involves the stitching of inert materials of silicone rubber or silastic sponge on to the sclera to push the ocular layers inwards, or injection of air into the vitreous to float the retinal tear upwards. These implants very occasionally find their way to the surface of the conjunctiva as foreign bodies.

There is no single type retinal detachment operation (Figs 77 & 78), and different retinal surgeons have different preferences which

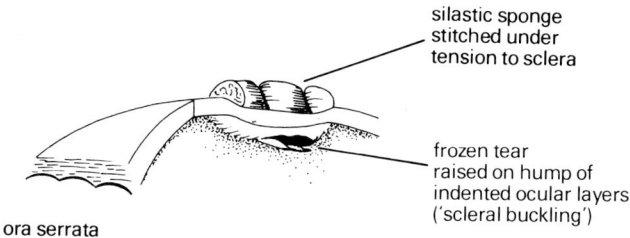

Fig. 77 One way to seal a retinal tear
Accuracy is clearly of paramount importance. Such accurate placement of the buckle is achieved with the indirect ophthalmoscope. Placement anywhere else will do nothing to seal the tear

they cannot always explain to others. However the success rate should be of the order of 95 per cent. Post-operative treatment is that of a surgically induced iritis which behaves no differently from any other iritis, namely local mydriatics and local corticosteroids. The eye should settle within a week, and the patient should be back to normal within a month.

Failure, apart from that due to frank surgical complication, follows retinal shrinkage for reasons that have not yet been wholly explained.

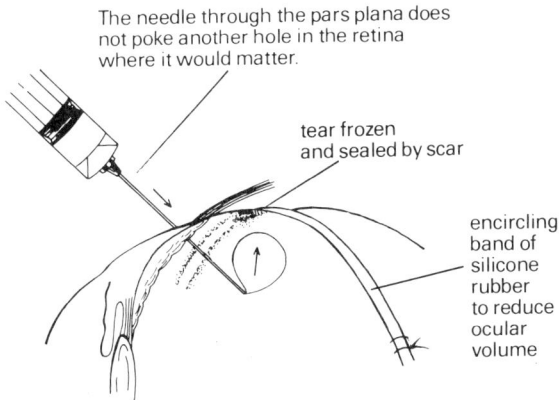

Fig. 78 Another way to seal a retinal tear
The air floats the detached retina upwards and absorbs in a few days

Retinal detachments not due to a retinal tear

Traction
The fibrous bands of diabetic retinopathy may pull the neuro-retina from its pigment layer. The same may follow trauma involving the vitreous cavity. Some of these are treatable surgically, sometimes by simple section of the traction band, though penetration of the vitreal cavity in a diabetic eye is more often followed by inflammatory resentment than by surgical cure.

Choroidal tumours
Primary or secondary malignant tumours of the choroid stimulate the collection of fluid beneath the adjacent retina (Fig. 79). If small enough, primary choroidal masses can be removed.

Inflammatory detachment
This is perhaps the rarest of all. Inflammation of the sclera or the choroid may flood the potential space with inflammatory fluid, the removal of which will depend on removal of the inflammation.

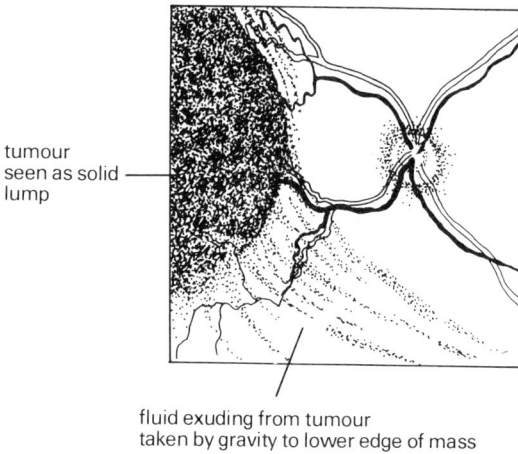

tumour
seen as solid
lump

fluid exuding from tumour
taken by gravity to lower edge of mass

Fig. 79 A retinal detachment due to a choroidal tumour

A retinal detachment is only an emergency when the central area of vision—the macula—is still intact. Detachment of the macula for no matter how brief a time will leave a mark on the central vision. Should operating facilities not be instantly available, then the patient should be positioned to allow the fluid to drain away by gravity from the macular area. With an upper detachment this will be the head down position, the other positions following logically from the ocular appearances. Should any doubt remain it is best to regard all detachments as ocular emergencies. An urgent ambulance journey is a small price to pay for intact central vision.

There is a disturbing post-script to all this. The eye in its emotive role as mirror of health and window to the soul has for centuries been the irresistible victim of our search for the elixir of life. The intra-ocular contents fortunately by their position evade any damaging attempts to improve them. The extra-ocular muscles, however, are available to be exercised beyond the limits of their natural movement on the assumption that, if strong is good, stronger is better. That they are already infinitely more powerful than they need be has not prevented mystics from promising a state of cosmic wellbeing at the extremes of every direction of gaze. All the world over the gullible are to be found rolling their eyes in search of Nirvana—fortunately for their reputation, in private.

Now it is a clinical impression that breaks, leading to retinal detachment, are frequently found in the retina just deep to these muscle insertions. And it is just conceivable that there might be some connection between these retinal breaks and extreme muscular traction movements in vulnerable eyes. Now the muscles are there, and presumably are intended to contract and relax. To ban all such actions would be patently absurd, but no more so than over-exercising them.

17

A miscellany of retinochoroidal disease

Retinoblastoma

This growth is fortunately as rare as it is malignant—occurring once in rather more than twenty thousand live births.

From its favourite site of origin in the posterior retina, it rapidly fills the vitreous with tumour seedlings. These deposits whiten the normally black pupil, and it is this feature rather than visual loss which catches parental notice.

Most cases present before the age of three, and there is a one in three chance that both eyes may be affected.

Treatment

Enucleation is obligatory for large tumours, but smaller ones may be attacked by a combination of radiotherapy and chemotherapy—both methods curing a large percentage of these unfortunate youngsters.

In known families the hereditary appears to be an autosomal dominant with 80 per cent penetrance. This means that half the children will carry the trait, and of this half four out of five will suffer the disease.

Where there is no family history it seems, however, that most cases are sporadic. More and more of these children survive to become parents themselves, and their offspring do not seem to demonstrate any dominant hereditary pattern.

Choroidal melanoma

This is the most common intra-ocular malignant growth—occurring in one eye usually after the age of 50. Because early symptoms are so slight, this tumour usually attracts attention when it is too big to submit to local removal. If ignored it would fill the cavity of the eye, blocking the aqueous drainage angle and causing an acute secondary glaucoma. Most often it is picked up as an incidental finding, or when the symptoms of creeping retinal detachment can no longer be ignored (see Fig. 79).

Distant metastases spread via the blood stream, landing classically in the liver, but like all classical patterns is a standard to be deviated from.

It is seen in the fundus as a solid mottled lump, frequently associated with an adjacent fluid retinal detachment carried by gravity into the lower part of the eye.

Management
If the mass be too large for local excision, then the current management is removal of the eye. However this is a moot point. Diagnosis of these lesions is sometimes extremely difficult, and a post-operative discovery that it was actually benign is not always a consolation to a patient who may have parted with a symptomless eye. Surgery itself may give a sudden impetus to blood borne spread, and the old adage, 'Beware of the one-eyed man with the large liver' must raise a question mark over the wisdom of enucleation in the first place.

Comparison of serial photographs over several months is perhaps the best compromise between instant enucleation and optimistic discharge from the eye hospital. Of course we must always exclude the possibility that what is taken for a primary malignant melanoma may in fact be a secondary tumour from a distant primary elsewhere.

Choroiditis (chorioretinitis)
While arising occasionally in the wake of other diseases, choroiditis is frequently an inflammation in its own right without any known cause. The traditional signs of inflammation collect in a patch in the posterior pole, resulting in exudation of inflammatory fluids into the vitreal cavity.

The result is malfunction of the affected retina, which is obscured by a suspension of inflammatory cells. Infections may continue to re-infect themselves, prolonging their appearance inside the eye. In the absence of re-infection, or indeed of any infection, choroidal inflammation will progress from acute exudation to scar formation over three to six weeks. Naturally this will result in destruction of the neuro-retina, pigment retina and choroid in an irregular and sporadic fashion (see Fig. 49).

The result will be non function of the affected retina, and should this be the macula, then of course central vision will be gone for ever. Should it be the peripheral retina then it may not be noticed. The final appearance will be that of a white sclera visible through a broken lacework of chorioretinal remnants—whorls and smudges of black pigment and fibrous tissue in a circumscribed patch surrounded by a normal red reflex.

Usually inflammation of the posterior cavity of the eye may come from no obvious source. Occasionally inflammation of the choroid and retina can result from infestation with toxoplasmosis—a protozoan parasite widespread in the animal kingdom.

As might be guessed treatment is generally of questionable value. Should the macula be threatened, then systemic corticosteroids may be justified to curtail as much as possible any irreparable damage to a fragile area.

Phakomatoses

These are included for completeness. A rare collection of lumps scattered throughout the body as well as the eye, and hovering uneasily between the title of genuine tumour and embryonic remnants, their names read like characters from a Lehar operetta: Von Recklinghausen, Von Hippel Lindau, Bourneville and Sturge-Weber.

Café au lait spots, skin tumours, intra-cranial gliomata, angiomatous malformations, sebaceous adenomata, and so on, will produce local damage and disorder wherever they alight. Unpredictable to some degree, fortunately they are as rare as they are untreatable.

Retinochoroidal degeneration and dystrophy

Senile macular degeneration

Perhaps the commonest of these degenerations, this condition occurs in a variety of guises, usually in the over 60s (Fig. 80). For some as yet unexplained reason, the retina subserving central vision begins to

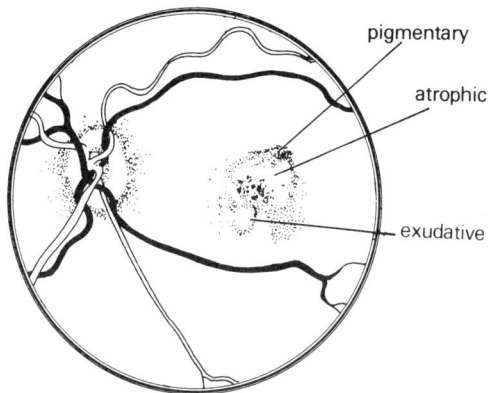

pigmentary

atrophic

exudative

This eye may have no central vision but it is not blind because the field is intact.

Fig. 80 Macular degeneration

Again a breach in the treaty of the layers. The final appearance depends on which layer dominates: it may be found in extreme degrees of progressive short sight disintegrate. Considering its complexity the wonder is that it does not do so earlier in life. Whatever layer primarily gives way, the end result is one or a blend of four things: macular atrophy, exposing the white sclera, exudation, abnormal pigmentation or frank haemorrhage, obscuring not only the scleral white but the choroidal red as well.

Occasionally a remote source of oedema into the macula can be identified by intravenous sodium flourescein and coagulated by the Laser. In the main, however, these degenerations progress mercilessly to total loss of central vision. The comfort is of course that it is only the central vision that is so affected. The field, in the absence of chronic glaucoma, which is itself common in that age group, will remain intact.

Myopia
Extremes of short sight produce extensive areas of chorioretinal thinning—as though not enough retina and choroid were available to cover so large an eye. Short sighted people on their own admission are a different breed from normal sighted, and generally tolerate visual disabilities unacceptable to their more normal sighted confrères. Even they, however, object when degeneration involves the macula, which it occasionally does, or when the thinned retina gives way as a retinal detachment, which it does with rather greater frequency. The latter is at least treatable.

Benign equatorial degeneration
Again in older age groups a fine spun interlacing pattern of dotted pigmentation encircles the globe around the equator. This might be seen at the extremes of gaze with the direct ophthalmoscope through the dilated pupil. The significance is the danger that casual observation may lead to a mistaken diagnosis of retinitis pigmentosa.

Retinitis pigmentosa
There is no more emotive condition than this. Beginning between the ages of six and twelve, and more common in men than women, this bilateral inherited malady leads to a total destruction of retinal function (Fig. 81).

A scatter of pigment clumps in the shape of bone corpuscles recalled from our histology days, creeps around the posterior pole of the retina just behind the equator. As the retina atrophies, so does the ability to see in the dark, with the natural onset of night blindness. This is then followed by progressive constriction of the visual field, until in the 50s only a few degrees of central vision are spared. This so-called tunnel vision, also occurring in chronic glaucoma, is visually very disabling and has prompted much so far fruitless research, and many expensive and trumpery remedies. Despite the impressive manipulation of polysyllabic chemicals in remote and picturesque clinics, there is no convincing evidence that any of them do more than introduce yet another alien poison to the system.

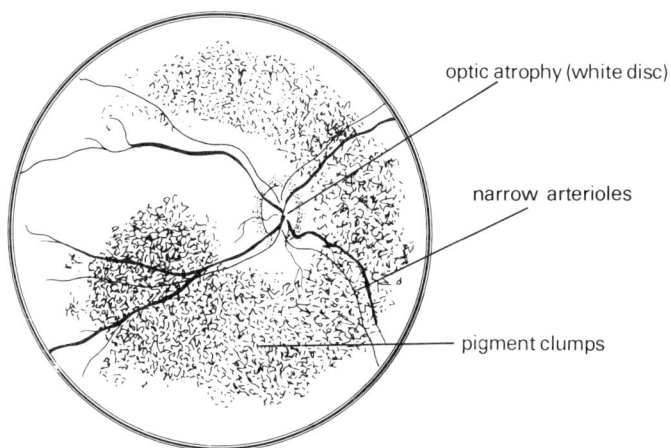

Fig. 81 Retinitis pigmentosa
    There are commoner causes of equatorial pigmentation

Albinism
The retinal pigment layer plays a vital function in the metabolism of visual pigments as well as absorbing excess of light. Its absence, recognisable before ophthalmoscopy, by the classic pale skin and bleached white hair of the Albino, can also be recognised by the appearance of the red reflex, not only through the pupil but through the atrophic iris as well.

Such eyes do not see well, not only because of absent necessary metabolites, but also because the existing retina is overwhelmed by the light presented. There are other familial progressive, and unfortunately untreatable chorio-retinal degenerations—whether called choroideraemia or gyrate atrophy—all result in night blindness and tunnel vision. Whether due to choroidal atrophy or retinal atrophy or both, is of little practical comfort to the patient, who just doesn't see well, and as the years go by will see even less.

18

Pupil reflexes and some common abnormalities

The pupil, which is the hole in the centre of the iris, is effectively a shutter which serves two purposes. Firstly it regulates the amount of light entering the eye. Secondly it constricts for near vision to allow a greater precision of near focus (Fig. 82).

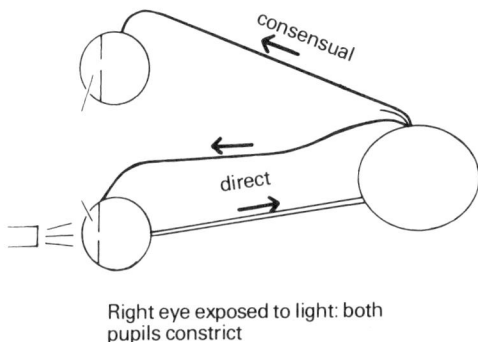

Right eye exposed to light: both
pupils constrict

Fig. 82 The reaction of the normal pupils
Both pupils constrict on exposure of one to a bright light. They also constrict when the eyes attempt near focus

The light reflex
This takes place at the level of the mid-brain, with a single inflow pathway travelling from the retina along the optic nerve and optic tract to the lateral geniculate body.

At the level of the mid-brain connection is made with the third nerve nucleus on each side to initiate the outflow impulse. This explains the existence of the direct and consensual reflex. Illumination of one eye will make both pupils constrict.

The near reflex
The inflow pathway, although the subject of many imaginative speculations, is unknown. It has however been suggested that contraction of the medial rectus muscles on convergence initiates the

ingoing stimulus. The outflow can be considered the same as that of the light reflex.

Inflow defect

Disturbance at any point along the inflow pathway eliminates or reduces the inflow stimulus along that side. This results in a diminished constriction of the pupil on the affected side (direct reflex) and on the opposite side (consensual reflex).

Outflow defect

Disturbance at any point along the outflow pathway will result in diminished constriction on the affected side, no matter which eye is illuminated.

The classic example of an inflow defect is retrobulbar neuritis, where the direct reflex on the affected side and the consensual reflex in the fellow eye is poorly sustained. Illumination of the fellow eye of course produces a normal response on both sides.

A third nerve palsy is the most extreme example of an outflow defect where the pupil is obstinately dilated, no matter which eye is exposed to light. Ptosis over an abducted depressed eye form the classic signs of a third nerve palsy, and we must assume that the cause is an intra-cranial aneurysm until this can be confirmed or disproved.

These reflexes must be provoked with a powerful light, and perhaps the commonest cause of a poorly sustained light reflex is a dying battery. And while we might ascribe a partial third nerve palsy to a host of unpleasant causes, dilatation of the pupil with Cyclopentolate, Tropicamide or Atropine is the most likely. It has not been unknown for a neurologist to be baffled by such a dilatation, and more baffled when a later examination reveals the pupil to be back to normal.

Sympathetic innervation

The pupil dilates under the action of the sympathetic fibres which pass up the cervical sympathetic chain to the dilator muscles of the iris. The pupils widening with emotion are a common device in romantic and horror fiction. This also explains why anxiety is so frequently a prelude to angle closure glaucoma.

Horner's syndrome

The pupils may be mildly different in size in normal people, but if a difference in pupil size is marked we must decide that one is either too small or the other too large.

Paralysis of the cervical sympathetic chain at its root in the neck can constrict the pupil on the affected side, and is classically caused by a space occupying lesion at the apex of the lung.

The Argyll Robertson pupil

This famous defect, associated with cerebral syphilis, results in a small irregular pupil that fails to respond to the strongest light. However it can be seen to respond to near focus, giving rise to comparison with student lodgings of a former generation as having accommodation but no light.

The Holmes-Adie pupil

The myotonic pupil, not associated with cerebral syphilis, is rather larger than normal, and although not responding promptly to light and accommodation, will do so eventually if given enough time, and it will take as long again to relax. Associated with loss of focus, and also with loss of tendon reflexes, it is perhaps more common in young women.

Constriction of such a pupil by Mecholyl in dilute concentrations that would have no effect on a normal pupil, passes from text book to text book as a mandatory element of diagnosis. It is generally in the text books that this remains, for by the time the unstable solution has been prised from the grasp of a reluctant pharmacist, its potency will have gone, and indeed so may have the patient, with the diagnosis accepted on clinical grounds alone.

Pinpoint pupils

Although the pupils of the morphine addict are well known to devotees of American television, perhaps the most likely reason is the use of Pilocarpine drops for chronic glaucoma. Advancing age has the same effect and in all cases both eyes are affected.

Other pupil distortions

An actual section of the pupil can be missing as in congenital coloboma, classically in the lower nasal quadrant. A surgical version of the same—a sector iridectomy through the 12 o'clock meridian—will be produced during a cataract extraction.

A blow on the eye can paralyse the pupil's sphincter, resulting in a traumatic mydriasis, and sometimes an iris prolapse. And of course acute glaucoma cannot exist without there being first a dilatation of the pupil.

The iris itself may be distorted by tumour formation, and if adhesions have followed an iritis sticking the iris to the lens, then an irregularly distorted pupil will result, and only the free margin will respond to light unless someone has already instilled atropine. The important thing is to know the classic pupil defects; all the others can be worked out from our list of aetiology. The reflexes are a natural part of the general cranial nerve examination. It is perhaps the briskness of their response rather than their starting point which is significant. A good rule in central nervous system disorders is that one isolated sign may be no sign at all.

19

Optic nerve head swellings

A small collection of disconnected conditions may result in a swollen, or apparently swollen, optic nerve head. Not all are significant, but all must be regarded so until proved safe. They divide into two groups:

Those presenting with visual symptoms.

Those presenting without visual symptoms (Fig. 83).

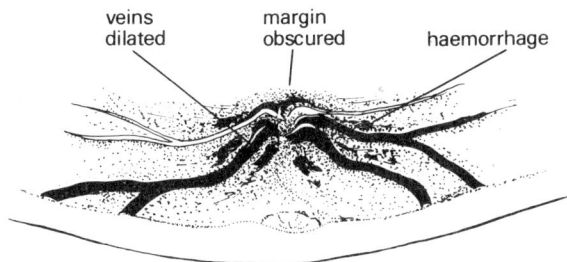

Fig. 83 The swollen optic disc
If papilloedema, there may be no visual loss. If papillitis (optic neuritis), there may be no vision

Those with visual symptoms

Optic neuritis
This is one of these names which flash to mind from student days without any accompanying flash of understanding. Inflammation from the optic nerve head, like inflammation anywhere else, can develop as a result of local or remote infection, but by far the highest proportion is due to demyelination, and most of these patients will go on to develop the general signs of multiple sclerosis.

The vision is grievously affected—central at first, and then the field. The pupil responds poorly to light and sustains this response even more poorly. Indeed so poor is the response that no dilating drop is required to see that the disc has lost its normal features:

1. *The margin is blurred.*
2. *The colour is more florid.*
3. *The cup may be reduced.*

The retinal vessels may be engorged.

Should this inflammation occur further back in the optic nerve, we call the condition *retrobulbar neuritis*, and a normal optic nerve head gives no hint of its presence.

Ischaemic optic neuropathy

Elderly patients with temporal arteritis especially, may suffer acute anoxia of the optic nerve head.

Vision will be reduced to absence of light perception. There will be no direct pupil reaction. The optic disc shows the following features: the margin will be blurred; the colour will be pale, and the disc swollen by an oedematous thickening, which obscures and fills in the optic cup.

The danger of temporal arteritis is that the second eye may follow suit with equal suddenness while the first eye is being pondered. A raised ESR indicates the need for systemic corticosteroids until an urgent temporal artery biopsy confirms or refutes the diagnosis.

Venous occlusion

Blockage of the central vein produces, predictably enough, a flood of haemorrhages through the retina together with oedema and swelling of the optic nerve head.

Visual loss, though severe, is never total. The pupil is correspondingly sluggish.

The disc will lose its normal margin.

The colour will be floridly red and haemorrhagic. No cup will be visible.

A faltering blood flow can be tipped into frank obstruction by chronic elevation of the intra-ocular pressure. The commonest cause of this elevation is chronic simple glaucoma, but the dramatic changes of venous occlusion would obscure the less dramatic signs of optic disc cupping. A normal disc in the fellow eye unfortunately does not guarantee that the pressure on that side is within acceptable limits.

The swollen disc without visual symptoms

Papilloedema

A choked optic nerve head is the classic sign of raised intra-cranial pressure. In itself it has no immediate effect on vision, and the patient will present with symptoms and signs quite remote from the eye. The cause remains unexplained. It is generally agreed that elevation of the cerebrospinal fluid pressure transmitted along the sheaths of the optic nerves is an initiating factor.

Thereafter, as a secondary phenomenon, the venous drainage from the eye becomes blocked and, more subtly still, there is some disturbance in the axoplasmic transport, allegedly resulting in white debris on the optic nerve head, and within its microcirculation. Whatever the exact mechanisms, this usually bilateral condition must be taken as a sign of raised intra-cranial pressure.

Not all such cases harbour cerebral tumours. Benign intra-cranial hypertension, a condition with a variety of associates, including the contraceptive pill, imitates a tumour so well that a full neurological examination is needed.

Systemic corticosteroids given for this are less unpleasant to tolerate than a sojourn in hospital.

The CAT (Computerised Axial Tomography) scan may reach this conclusion on an outpatient basis without the infernal apparatus which used to preface surgery on the brain.

The vision is usually normal.

The pupils will also be normal unless the cause of the raised pressure has also affected the visual pathways.

The margin of the optic disc is blurred and concealed.

The colour is florid, the disc substance swells and diminishes the cup.

The retinal veins may be engorged and a few local haemorrhages complete the picture. These are never as dramatic as in venous occlusion, where the visual loss would make a diagnosis of papilloedema impossible.

Pseudopapilloedema
Small crowded (long sighted) eyes have small crowded discs where there is not enough room for all the normal appearances to take their rightful place. There may be some doubts about the margin, the colour will be red. There will be no cup.

There will also be no symptoms, but there will be great anxiety when this chance finding has been made.

Should any doubt exist, it is possible to dispel this doubt. A yellow dye (sodium fluorescein), already celebrated for its use on the cornea, if injected into one of the arm veins can be traced as it flows through the eye and will demonstrate the presence or absence of abnormal swellings of the optic nerve head.

The important distinction between the first group of conditions and the second is that the first are all brought to our attention by some visual catastrophe. The second might not have been brought at all if someone had followed the ritual of examination, and looked at the optic nerve heads even though such an examination was not necessarily indicated.

20

Childhood eye problems

Most of these have already been examined in other chapters, but there are a few that more naturally assemble under the heading of age than of anatomy.

The problem with little patients is to get near enough for an adequate look at eyes whose alleged malfunction is always the subject of a second-hand history.

Infantile glaucoma

The anterior chamber in the developing baby is full of embryonic tissue that normally disappears, but sometimes fails to. Should this tissue block the drainage angle then of course the intra-ocular pressure must rise. The infantile sclera, however, stretches under this raised pressure, producing a large eye which waters, dislikes the light, has a hazy cornea and which, if neglected, will eventually fail to see (Fig. 84).

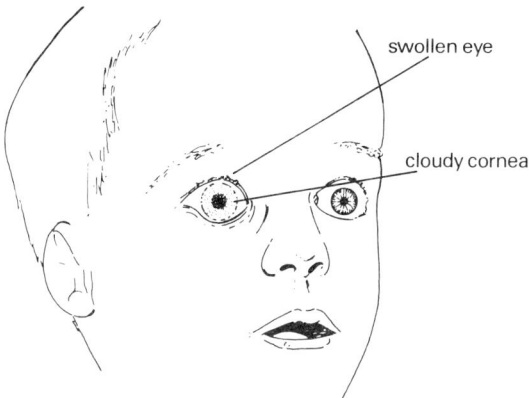

Fig. 84 Congenital glaucoma (buphthalmos)

It must of course be distinguished from a large normal cornea where there is a total absence of all other signs. It should be remembered that the two-year-old cornea is already adult size, giving children those magnificent and apparently huge eyes that excite a bitter sweet regret in withered adults who contemplate their own childhood portraits.

Treatment of infantile glaucoma is surgical—a simple goniotomy with a needle to clear away abnormal tissue from a normal angle. Normal drainage and normal vision should follow.

However should the angle also be abnormal as part of an inherited defect, then an external drainage operation will be required. These tend not to succeed because the only healthy thing about these eyes is their fibrotic response to anything so outrageous as a deliberate surgical fistula. Visual decline sadly then is relentless.

Iritis and Still's disease

Iritis complicates both adult and juvenile rheumatism, though tragically the complications are infinitely more damaging in children, because the iritis does not resolve. It smoulders into a destructive condition that poisons the eye as the years go by. Corticosteroids, both local and systemic, only delay the inevitable decline into cataract, secondary glaucoma, failed operations for secondary glaucoma, band-shaped scars across the front of the cornea and finally visual collapse. Fortunately it is as rare as it is untreatable.

Coloboma

If it is remembered that the eyeball and the lower lid have a single 'seam of union' running from the optic disc forwards along the lower nasal meridian, then failure of this seam to close perfectly is called a coloboma (Fig. 85). It may range from a negligible notch in the eyelid to a total absence of everything but sclera along the line of failed closure. No treatment is indicated except when a retinal detachment complicates the issue.

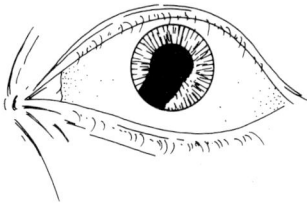

Fig. 85 Iris coloboma
The gap in the iris may extend along what should be the normal line of closure as far as the optic disc

Conjunctivitis, Spring catarrh, squint, retinoblastoma, Coat's disease, and a host of rare malformations complete the picture of childhood eye disease.

The problems differ from adults only in the amount of effort required to coax children into co-operation, and this can be almost a veterinary problem.

Examination under anaesthesia may be required, but first must always be justified. However it is tragic to miss a treatable detachment because of everyone's reluctance to resort to anaesthesia. As with all other branches of medicine, the skill lies in knowing when to proceed with further investigation and when to reassure. A fair attempt at the examination ritual, with the pupil dilated, should go a long way to make this decision an easy one.

21

Painless loss of vision

Any physical disorder from the eyelids back to the occipital cortex can give rise to visual loss of one sort or another. The task of finding out exactly which disorders might seem hopeless, when in theory so many of them lie within the skull. It may seem more hopeless still when we contemplate the entire visual pathway, trusting that some diagnostic flourish will emerge. Fear of making the wrong diagnosis may turn this metaphysical speculation into inertia.

The first step to the right diagnosis is to examine the eye in the same way every time. The second step is to recognise that this visual pathway is not all of a piece, and the third step is to realise that common disorders are common, and there are not that many of them (Fig. 86).

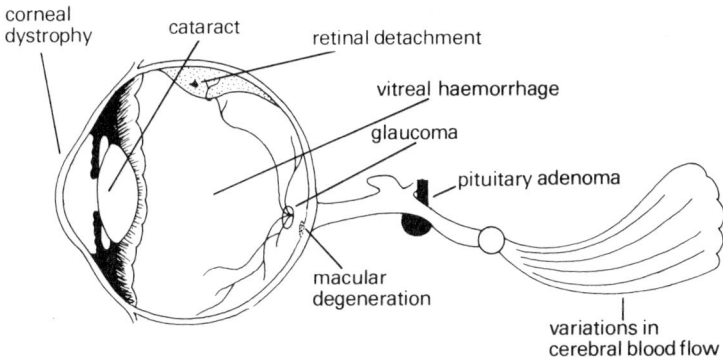

Fig. 86 Painless loss of vision
If the examination ritual be observed so will the diagnostic signs

We must first decide if the visual loss is real or apparent. The latter is surprisingly frequent, and people occasionally take umbrage that they should actually be expected to know how well they saw before seeking a consultation. It is also worth repeating that most judge the state of their eyes by the state of their central vision. Gradual creeping field loss may cause no concern until it involves the macula, when allegations of sudden visual impairment will bring the patient up to hospital in some urgent distress.

The visual apparatus anterior to the optic chiasma produces vision and visual symptoms in one eye alone; the portion behind the chiasma produces vision and visual symptoms in the binocular field of the opposite side—a concept too much for most people who tend to think of one eye—one side.

Dramatic vascular accidents and slow degenerations are more likely at a time when age is beginning to make off with the faculties. In the middle years unsuspected hypertension or diabetes may shatter those who think they are fit and well, and suddenly find that they are neither. In the healthy young we should be thinking in terms of congenital defects, injuries and episodes of demyelination.

The common disorders tend to be found in one eye or both—affecting either the clear media—the cornea, the lens or the vitreous—the optic nerve, the retinal vessels, the macula or the peripheral retina—in other words the structures that are looked at anyway during the routine system of examination.

The pinhole disc and confrontation test will indicate what and how severe the complaint might be. The cornea, the pupil and the depth of the anterior chamber might even give the answer before we proceed to dilate the pupil for an ophthalmoscopic examination.

Cataract

The most common opacity in the transparent structures is cataract, whether senile of congenital. It will appear as a silhouette against the red reflex to an ophthalmoscope held 8 to 12 in away from the eye. Because someone has senile cataract this does not mean that he has not got chronic simple glaucoma or macular degeneration or indeed all three. The patient's response to visual testing should have given the clues (see Fig. 56).

Not all opacities are due to cataract. The vitreous may fill with blood from diabetic haemorrhage, or inflammatory cells from a chorioretinitis, and both should appear in silhouette against the red reflex.

Chronic simple glaucoma

The optic disc, the next structure in the line for scrutiny, will show vertical extension of the central cup. Because to most people central vision is the only vision, they may be quite unaware of gradual erosion of their field, ascribing any slight defects to the inevitable decline of age. Chronic glaucoma is usually picked up during routine testing for spectacles, and sadly not always then. Like the tests for the pork tapeworm, imperfect examination is probably worse than no examination at all, for a patient may be allowed to go blind while convinced that he is not. The whole point of ophthalmic examination is to ensure the detection of treatable disease. Most of these will draw attention to themselves. Not so glaucoma, which is recognisable to the patient only when the field has gone (see Fig. 64).

Senile macular degeneration

We now move to the macula where the other common degenerative process is found. As its name implies, it occurs commonly in the twilight of life and, acting as the reverse of glaucoma, it damages the central vision while leaving the field intact. Central vision may be removed beyond the point of correction, no matter what optical device be employed. Pigmentary atrophy or haemorrhage or frank scarring affecting the macula alone, can be seen only through the dilated pupil (see Fig. 80).

This degeneration has the unfortunate habit of striking people whose brains are otherwise rather lively, but as long as the hand movement field remains intact and unimpaired by chronic glaucoma, then there is no reason for these people to go blind. *The difference between loss of central vision and loss of all vision is enormous.* It can bring great comfort to those with macular degeneration to remind them of just how enormous the difference is, and it can bring greater comfort still to keep things that way.

Hypertension and diabetes

Hard yellow exudates in a star figure commonly reduce macular function in hypertension. The deeper exudates of diabetes, with no rigid shape imposed upon them by the nerve fibre layer, spread in irregular islands destroying the deep retinal layers with a similar result. The general signs of hypertensive or diabetic retinopathy should then lead us to measure the blood pressure and test the urine for sugar (see Figs. 51 & 53).

The retinal vessels

Occlusion of the central retinal vein

The fundal picture is of the stormy sunset retina, where the turmoil of flame haemorrhages, swollen veins and retinal oedema is unforgettable in an eye that will have lost a fair degree of central vision. Increased blood viscosity and general vascular disease must be excluded. The raised intra-ocular pressure of chronic glaucoma may reduce the venous flow to the point of stasis, and indeed must be assumed to have done so until proved blameless by formal measurement of the intra-ocular pressure (see Fig. 55A & B).

Occlusion of the central retinal artery
The creamy white retina where the only visible red reflex is through the macula (the cherry red spot) is perhaps a less dramatic appearance than its venous counterpart. The visual loss, however, is more dramatic and usually total. A combination of hypertension and arteriosclerosis may be at fault, but temporal arteritis must be assumed in the over 60s until ruled out by a low erythrocyte sedimentation rate (ESR). If the ESR be raised, it is obligatory to prescribe systemic corticosteroids and remove a segment of the temporal artery for biopsy as a matter of some urgency (see Fig. 54).

Optic neuritis
A swollen optic nerve head with gross visual loss means demyelination, especially in the younger age groups. In older people the acute ischaemia of temporal arteritis is more likely.

Many students and elderly doctors pursue their career unaware that optic neuritis and retrobulbar neuritis are in fact the same condition, differing only in where they strike the optic nerve head. Optic neuritis will be visible as a swollen disc. Retrobulbar neuritis, on the other hand, is one of these conditions where the patient sees nothing and the doctor sees nothing. Both conditions are likely to follow demyelination, and most will go on to develop multiple sclerosis if followed up long enough (see Fig. 83).

Tobacco amblyopia
Addicts of heavy black Cavendish, especially those who flavour their addiction with hard spirits, may over the years begin to lose their central vision. Failing red/green discrimination and eventual optic atrophy only confirm a suspicion that the history should have already raised. Cyanide from the pipe overwhelms the enzyme system that in normal circumstances would have turned it into harmless thiocyanate. This pitiless decline of macular function can be halted by parenteral hydroxocobalamin. A change in personal habits, with alternative sources of calories, may contribute to the patient's general wellbeing.

If the examination so far has produced no signs, we must now turn to the peripheral retina, where significant though less common pathology may lie.

Retinal detachment
This is recognised by a rippling grey reflex which obscures the normal

red one. If arising from the upper retina, its impact is usually sudden. However, detachments from the lower retina may not be recognised until they have affected the macula—another example of people judging their vision by the centre alone. Such a detachment may happen as a result of congenital weakness at its peripheral edge, or because of a long forgotten injury. Gravity and a healthy vitreous will impede the development of the detachment, as well as the patient's awareness of what is happening (see Fig. 75).

Choroidal melanoma
The presentation is not unexpectedly that of a creeping retinal detachment—but unfortunately one with a malignant basis in the choroid, and usually in the fifth decade of life (see Fig. 79).

Intra-cranial disease
Disorders inside the head affecting the visual pathways will generally come to our notice because they are affecting something else as well.

Tumours will as a rule produce headache and papilloedema before they produce loss of vision. But just occasionally an intra-cranial aneurysm or a pituitary adenoma may break this rule. They can both present with visual defects—the former apparently inexplicable and the latter all too readily ascribed to a 'glaucomatous process', where the intra-ocular pressure, for some unclarified reason, remains defiantly normal.

Variations in the blood flow by their very nature vary, but become significant only when the circulation is already trembling on the brink of insufficiency. Unaccustomed exercise can deflect an already sparse cerebral blood flow elsewhere. Any rapid changes in posture, the head reaching a new position before its blood supply, must give rise to many symptoms, of which visual loss is but one. With an even more compromised circulation such symptoms can occur without any movement at all. In most of them, the visual fields classically constrict, clouding in grey from the periphery, and clearing in the reverse direction.

With progressive lesions, the visual loss tends to be progressive also. With fluctuating volumes of blood flowing through the head, although the vision may go from time to time, it also tends to come back again.

SUMMARY

Almost all causes of painless visual loss will occur anterior to the optic chiasma, and a few simple questions can confirm this. Thereafter the search is simplified by an awareness of what is likely, in what sort of person.

The degenerative disorders are clearly more common in those who have lived long enough for such things to happen. Because they develop gradually their onset in one eye may not be noticed until the other eye has begun to suffer the same thing. It should be remembered that anyone old enough to suffer one of the degenerative disorders is also old enough to develop the others, and indeed may have done so already.

Vascular accidents are more likely in those whose circulation has passed a lifetime through it. Because they are sudden, they tend to strike one eye at a time, but should the underlying condition be left unchecked, the other eye may follow with equal rapidity.

Congenital defects will demonstrate themselves rather early in life if they are significant. They also tend to affect both eyes.

Trauma, by its very nature, is sporadic, although the eyes are very vulnerable to deliberate assault when rapid punching or kicking may produce identical lesions on each side. Hypertension, which might be considered the chronic glaucoma of general medicine, can wreak its havoc unsuspected before showing its hand and trumping the eye with a venous or arterial occlusion, or the brain with a stroke.

The important thing is to work through the simple examination ritual—alert to what might have happened, ready to change our minds if it is apparent that something unexpected has happened, and continually aware that in the elderly many things may have happened. The unchanging ritual of examination will ensure that whatever has happened is not missed.

Trauma

Injuries, no matter where they strike the body, have two aspects. The first and obvious one is the instant damage. The second is the possible long term complication, either at the site of injury or at a more distant site.

Apart from a few well defined conditions demanding urgent specialist attention, anyone familiar with the craft of suturing can attend to most ocular injuries. They are skin lacerations usually, and 'ocular' only because they lie around the eyes.

Injuries become 'specialist ocular' in four main categories, and the only equipment necessary to evaluate the damage is a good torch, whilst the other eye may serve as a normal control.

INTRA-OCULAR FOREIGN BODY

In any violence involving the eye, a foreign body within the globe should always be suspected. Fragments of steel from a hammer or chisel, or pieces of shattered windscreen are common culprits. It is always wise to ask if anything was travelling fast enough to penetrate the eye. However the inability to judge the value of goggles when hammering, or seat belts when driving may extend to the velocity of possible intruders.

Close examination of the eyeball may show an entry point, iris distortion being a helpful guide (Fig. 87). But a fragment entering the limbus could leave the eye looking entirely normal until its ill effects become obvious some time later.

If an eye hospital is close at hand then referral is the correct approach. However in remoter districts a radiograph of the orbit is a useful preliminary. Absence of orbital opacities could save a needless journey; whereas a positive demonstration of these could save the eye.

Intra-ocular metal fragments left long enough in situ will oxidise and deposit metal salts throughout the globe. Ferrous metals may come out easily with a magnet, but other metals like copper require forceps removal. The lens, indifferent to the exact nature of the penetrating agent, may develop a cataract if the foreign body has damaged it on the way in.

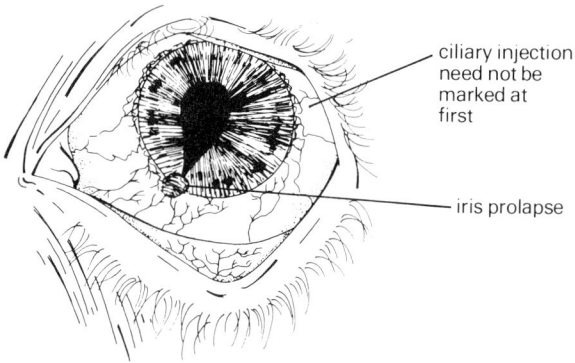

Fig. 87 Rupture of the cornea
Intra-ocular structures on the outside may mean something alien on the inside

DIRECT EYEBALL INJURY

This may be lacerating, blunt or chemical.

Lacerations
Lacerations are easily recognised. It is vital to avoid anything that might raise the intra-ocular pressure, and hence empty the eye of its contents.

Blunt injury
The imagination can supply all likely agents, but ball games and fisticuffs must rank high on the list. The front of the eye may fill with blood—hyphaema—which is recognised when the turbidity has settled, by a fluid level (see Fig. 48).

A blow sufficient to cause such a haemorrhage may well have caused a silent rupture of the globe as well. A hyphaema filling the entire anterior chamber can block the drainage angle and cause an acute secondary glaucoma. If not cleaned out soon, the blood may stain the cornea. Later developments from blunt trauma may show in after years. Chronic secondary glaucoma can follow fibrosis of the drainage angle, or retinal tears sustained from the original blow can bring about a retinal detachment at any time—so long after, in fact, that the connection may not be suspected (Fig. 88). A lens that survives dislocation may not survive cataract formation.

Chemical injury
The range could be bewildering, but strong acids or alkalis are

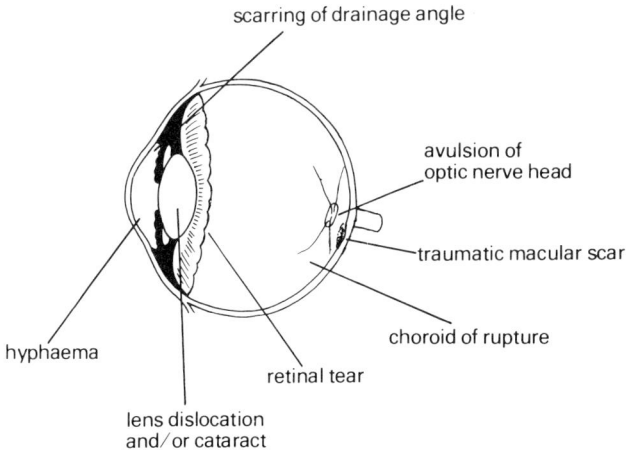

Fig. 88 Trauma can produce one, or a blend of all these conditions, not always immediately

particularly popular with bank raiders and have always been familiar on the industrial scene.

Instant washing out with water must be the first move, with the emphasis on speed.

Both chemicals can cause lethal damage. They will distort the eyelids, causing them to adhere to the eye, turn in the lashes, opacify the cornea and scarify the drainage angle. Alkali injuries are the more sinister in that they seep deeper into the eye, causing more complicated disturbance than do acids, whose coagulating action limits their penetration.

EYELID INJURY

There are two situations demanding specialist attention within 24 hours (Fig. 89):

1. Laceration involving the lid margin.
2. Laceration involving the lower canaliculus.

Unless the lid margins are accurately opposed, a notch at the injury site can result in permanent intractable watering, not to mention what exposure or ingrowing lashes can do to the corneal epithelium.

The watering that follows neglected canalicular injuries is even more distressing—the more so since early surgery might have cured a condition which later surgery almost never can.

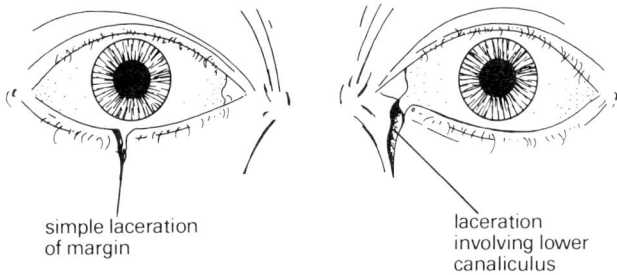

simple laceration
of margin

laceration
involving lower
canaliculus

Fig. 89 Laceration of the lid margins
   Top priority is restoration of the alliance of the anterior segment and of
preserving a channel of communication along the canaliculus

ORBITAL INJURY

Blow out fracture of the orbital floor is a popular weekend injury (Fig.
90), often sustained when the victim's subjective awareness is not at
its best. A savage blow forces the orbital contents into the maxillary
sinus, where the eye muscles will be trapped by the bony fragments.
The tethered eye will not move either upwards or downwards, and if
the condition is neglected, never will.

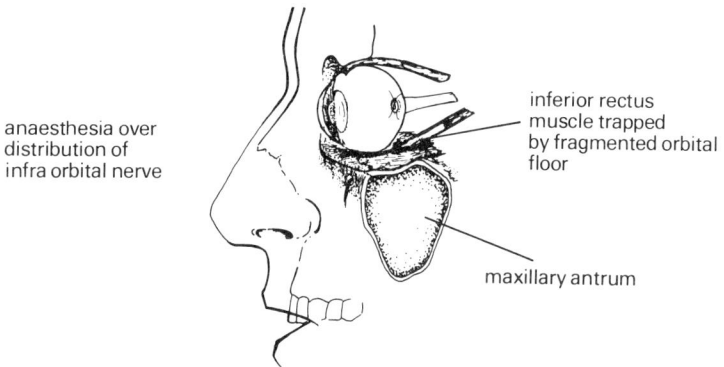

anaesthesia over
distribution of
infra orbital nerve

inferior rectus
muscle trapped
by fragmented orbital
floor

maxillary antrum

Fig. 90 Blow out fracture of the orbital floor
   Trauma sufficient to smash the bones may do something similar to the eye

   Diplopia would be recognised by the patient if other symptoms
were not occupying his attention.
   The first step to diagnosis is to consider it likely from the type of
injury. Tethered eye movements and loss of sensation over the
distribution of the infra-orbital nerve between the orbital margin and
the lip are classical signs. Settling oedema may demonstrate that the
eye has sunk rather in comparison with its fellow.

It should be remembered that damage severe enough to smash the bone may have also smashed the eye. If the swollen lids have to be forced open to permit a glimpse of the eye, a comparison with its fellow for corneal clarity and anterior chamber equality may set the mind at rest, at least in the short term.

Radiographic examination will confirm or refute any clinical impression.

It is necessary to elevate the contents of the orbit and keep them in position with a plate of silicone rubber to make good the defect in the orbital floor.

Since many of these cases finally come to court, some attempt at measuring visual acuity makes the medical evidence more convincing and may make all the difference to any subsequent damage settlements.

Sympathetic ophthalmitis

A penetrating eye injury can give rise to many troubles, but this condition is its most dreadful complication. In the first two weeks after an injury, especially one involving the lens and ciliary body, circulating antibodies to normal eye tissue may be formed. These antibodies, failing to recognise the eyes as 'self', may then attack both of them, and they will respond with a smouldering, destructive, inflammatory process.

Clearly it is essential to recognise the danger signals and remove the injured eye before the fellow eye becomes involved—for then it would be too late.

In practice, it can be assumed that there is no danger during the first two weeks when the damaged eye should be settling from the trauma and the restorative surgery. If it continues to settle, all is well.

However, should the eye flare up again, then the renewed pain, watering and redness must warn the doctor to consider enucleation.

Although these dismaying decisions are usually taken within three to four weeks of an accident, no perforated eye is ever wholly safe. It is, therefore, wise to regard with caution any casual inflammatory episodes that may affect such an eye.

SUMMARY

Damage to the eyelid risks the integrity of its margin or the potency of the lower canaliculi. Injury to the globe apart from its obvious features may in the long term result in cataract, chronic secondary glaucoma, and retinal detachment.

An intra-ocular foreign body is always possible no matter how convincing may be the history to the contrary.

A blow out fracture of the orbit may not be apparent until the oedema of the facial injury has disappeared.

Any penetrating eye injury including surgery can give rise to sympathetic ophthalmitis.

23

Skin diseases and the eye

The eye may share in disturbances of the skin because the lids and lashes, conjunctiva, cornea and lens all derive from the surface ectoderm. Skin disturbances are known as dermatoses. When they affect the eye the names may change but the pathology does not.

Sebaceous gland overactivity
Misbehaviour of these glands on the face is the plague of teenagers who base their happiness on a flawless complexion and fail to see other qualities hidden behind a mask of scars and pustules. The Meibomian glands, as such glands in the eyelids are called, can act independently of their counterparts on the face. A frothy emulsion of oil and tears collects across the lid margins and the lashes—a fertile breeding ground for low grade infection.

When it occurs on the scalp we call it dandruff, and when on the eyelashes there is no reason why we should not call it dandruff of the eyelashes. Unfortunately the toxic agents used to rid the scalp of its scurf are not so easily applicable in the presence of a delicate cornea, where they may create a fresh ocular condition for which there is no effective remedy.

Rosacea
The name suggests hyperaemia which forms a background for pustules, papules and dilated blood vessels—classically distributed over the forehead, the nose and the cheeks. The distribution may spread to the conjunctiva and the cornea, with resultant corneal scars.

Oral Tetracycline tablets 250 mg twice daily for two months, have proved to be very successful in suppressing the condition, both in the skin and in the eye. Local emollient drops may add to the ocular comfort.

Infective dermatoses
Bacteria whether staphylococci or streptococci can multiply pathologically on the skin as anywhere else. The former limit

themselves to folliculitis, but the latter may spread through the skin as erysipelas and cellulitis. Both require prompt treatment with systemic and local antibiotics.

Eczema

The acute reaction is characterised by erythema and oedema. It is considered to be an allergic response, although to what is not always evident. Ophthalmic preparations of course produce such lesions around the eye, and the first step to relief of symptoms is to stop the offending medication.

Atopic eczema

The signs of eczema are augmented because the patient, in an attempt to produce the irritation, adds to it by rubbing. The condition becomes of ophthalmic interest by the development of cataract at an age when such an event should not happen. Predictably it is called dermatogenous cataract.

The bullous dermatoses

Erythema multiforme

This bullous disorder produces characteristic round target lesions on the palms and the soles. The causes include drug sensitivity and viral infections, and in its most severe form—Stevens-Johnson's syndrome—the mucous membranes are involved and this brings the condition into the realms of rare conjunctivitis.

As a sensitivity reaction the eye condition should respond in some way to local corticosteroids.

Benign mucous membrane pemphigoid

Called benign because it does not produce death, pemphigoid is anything but when it comes to the mucous membranes of the mouth and eyes. Shrinkage of the conjunctiva has devastating effects on corneal health and ocular mobility. It is included in this text because of its havoc and not because of its frequency.

Radiation

Those fortunate enough to stretch naked or near naked on the beaches of Southern France may well suffer sunburn. Its appearance is too well known to need description and the makers of bronzing lotions prosper greatly from our desire to risk it. Ultraviolet radiation to the front of the cornea produces a rather less pleasing result. Superficial pinpoint erosions—punctate keratitis—no different from that of a welding flash or from snow blindness, produce intense pain and watering, and diminution of vision. Classically symptoms appear some hours after exposure and persist for some days after the temperature has dropped. The corneal epithelium will recover if allowed to, behind closed eyelids. The temptation to remove the symptoms with local anaesthetic drops on a long term basis is probably actionable and will certainly produce more signs on an even longer term basis.

The erythematous dermatoses

Lupus erythematosus swarming across the face in a butterfly pattern is a systemic disorder—one of the so-called collagen diseases. These collagen disorders may affect the eye and do so by producing ischaemia. At the corneal margin this would appear as necrotic ulceration. In the retina new vessel formation and haemorrhage differ little from the effects of diabetes.

Scleroderma

Our knowledge alas extends only to a description of this condition, which results in hardening of the skin with ischaemic necrosis of the deeper tissues. The eyelids and conjunctiva may succumb to this process, with predictable effects on the globe.

To complete our aetiological list, congenital and hereditary vascular disturbances may affect the eye, but are not really part of a general skin condition. Trauma, too, can produce awful damage, but it is dermatological only in that the skin or its associates happen to be first in the line for injury.

Basal cell carcinoma of the eyelids brings us on to more familiar ground, and has to be differentiated from simple warts, cutaneous horns and mollusca contagiosa.

Pigmented lesions of the skin, deriving from melanocytes, form into four main groups with endless subdivisions. Lesions may be circumscribed, widespread, flat or raised, and are perhaps less significant in the African than they might be in a Scandinavian. In general terms they are best left well alone, and any alteration in shape, size or general appearance should be referred to an expert in such matters. Benign lesions may spontaneously become malignant, or may be helped on their way in that direction by ill-advised excision.

Although this must appear to be a disconnected catalogue, the effects of it on the eye need not differ from any other ophthalmic problem. The eye is still an organ of vision, and the ritual of examination should remain unchanged. Management is very much the same as the treatment of general skin disorders, except that we are prevented from using the more exuberant remedies lest we produce more fearful eye problems than we started with.

24

Proptosis

When the available space in the orbit ceases to be adequate to contain the eyeball as well as the orbital contents, then the eye with only the eyelids offering resistance will advance to appear prominently through the eyelid aperture. We call this condition proptosis (Fig. 91).

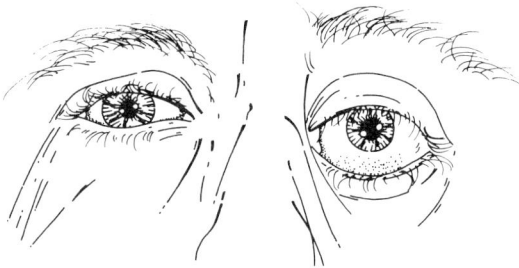

Fig. 91 Proptosis
Particularly threatened are the exposed cornea and the compressed optic nerve

Another name—exophthalmos—means very much the same thing but has tended to be reserved for proptosis due to thyroid disease when the orbital contents change not only their size but their character as well.

Dangers to the eye
There are two basic dangers. Long term compression of the optic nerve at the apex of the orbit can squeeze away its function as well as the normal colour of the optic nerve head, with diminishing vision and optic atrophy.

At the front, the eyelids fail to protect the cornea where the resultant desiccating exposure will produce superficial ulcers which, deepening through the sub-epithelial membrane (Bowman's), will permanently scar the affected areas.

Aetiology
A wide reaching collection of disease processes from the blood

dyscrasias to simple trauma can fill the orbital space with unhealthy or alien tissues. In practice, fortunately, the permutation reduces to a small workable collection—the most common being thyroid disease which, contrary to popular belief, may be unilateral in some 20 per cent of cases.

Symptoms

A mass within the orbit, no matter what its cause, may distort vision by pressing upon the eye. It may push the globe beyond the capacity of the muscles to maintain binocular vision. It may cause pain. It may expose the cornea with resultant watering. It will certainly produce a cosmetic defect. Once again, here is an example of widely different disease processes converging on the same clinical condition, using up all the available symptoms without particularly leading us to a certain diagnosis.

Examination

Deflection of the eye to one side would suggest a local mass—for example, a lacrimal gland tumour. Simple advance of the globe (axial proptosis), while it may follow a diffuse infiltration of the orbit, may also result from an optic nerve glioma. Thyroid disease is popularly associated with prominent eyes. Perhaps not so well known, restoration of the euthyroid state may, in fact, be associated with even more prominent eyes.

It was alleged that a thyroid stimulating hormone somehow also stimulated exophthalmos. This old explanation will not do now. However, what will do is not yet clear. Other substances with the names of long-acting thyroid stimulator or exophthalmos producing hormones are now blamed for their ill-effect on the eyes. Research keeps turning up a daunting catalogue of new and complexly named rivals and the proptosis continues indifferent to their discovery.

Retraction of the upper lid exaggerating the eyeball protrusion is a classic distinguishing feature of thyroid induced proptosis (Fig. 92). In the general flutter of sympathetic overactivity, the autonomic levator of the eyelid acts independently of its fellow. When the thyroid is not involved the upper eyelid tends not to be involved either.

Mucopolysaccharides deposited within the orbit and within the extra-ocular muscles push the eye forward and limit the ability of the muscles to maintain normal movements. Occasionally an oedematous conjunctiva may herniate and strangulate through tight eyelids.

A confident clinical diagnosis of thyroid disease is not always supported by abnormal blood levels of the various thyroid factors. It is at this point that search for another cause must begin. These might be

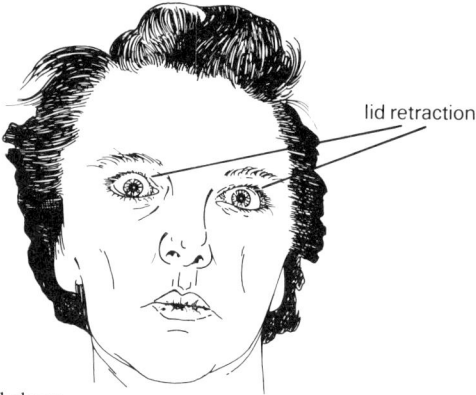

Fig. 92 Exophthalmos
Proptosis due to thyroid disease. Lid retraction augments the corneal exposure.
Infiltration of the extra-ocular muscles restricts their action

limited at the start to a full blood count and orbital X-ray films which
sometimes demonstrate bony erosion or widening of the optic
foramina. A collection of negative findings at this point leaves us
impaled on a diagnostic fork. Should we observe a proptosed eye
without a diagnosis or threaten the same eye by searching for one—the
biopsy of which may leave a nerve palsy in its track and produce a
nightmare smudge of tissues for the histologist to equivocate over.
There is much to be said for doing nothing, measuring regularly the
lack of change in both types of vision, corneal exposure and the optic
nerve head.

When increasing symptoms and signs make a diagnosis an urgent
necessity, then the CAT scan may provide enormous information
about the diagnosis and the orbital contents without damaging them.

Pseudo tumour
This uncommon unilateral grumbling granulomatous inflammation
may be mistaken for a neoplasm. If a biopsy be dared, it may
demonstrate some ambiguous differences from other more lethal
disorders. Resolution with high doses of systemic corticosteroid may
produce the same diagnosis by inference as well as a clinical
improvement without recourse to the knife.

Proptosis in children
Rhabdomyosarcoma is the most common malignancy found in an age
group when a malignant cause is the most likely.

Acute proptosis

Orbital cellulitis
This acute infection of the orbit, either as a blood borne disorder or as

a result of an adjacent sinusitis, results in all the local signs of inflammation as well as a systemic fever.

Cavernous sinus thrombosis

This rare and devastating bilateral catastrophe produces gross venous congestion and disturbance of the third, fourth, fifth and sixth cranial nerves which traverse the wall of the sinus on their way to the orbit.

The patient will be clearly prostrated by a severe illness and this is no time to debate trifles at length by the bedside. As both conditions are fortunately rare, it is not always easy to stand firm upon classical signs because they do not happen often enough to be classical; however, a unilateral condition with normal pupils in a reasonably well though fevered patient should make the distinction of orbital cellulitis from the more severely disturbing cavernous sinus thrombosis.

Management

The aim must be to preserve both the eye and life though in childhood malignancy neither of these is always possible. The cause should be removed but if it cannot then its ill-effects should be curbed. Long term function, of course, means the passage of light normally through a transparent cornea to a retina served by a healthy optic nerve.

At a simple level, corneal exposure may be soothed and indeed treated with artificial tears or by small plastic procedures to narrow the palpebral fissure. Diplopia due to muscle palsies does not always respond to surgical alteration of their position because the muscles themselves are diseased. A black patch over either eye may remove the symptoms and at the end of the day may be more effective than surgery. At a higher level the threat of gross corneal exposure or optic nerve compression may require a neurosurgeon to unroof the orbit.

Thereafter we must always balance the danger of the condition against the danger of the investigation. Many such eyes remain unchanged for years, defying all attempts at a diagnosis while the patient's survival demonstrates how wise it was in the first place to leave well alone.

25

Flashing lights

The sensation of lights flashing where there are no lights at all means that something is disturbing the visual pathway. This section of the brain runs from the neural retina along the optic nerve, the optic tract by the mid brain and backwards into the visual cortex, passing through the temporal and parietal lobes on the way. These visual parts of the brain are so specialised that they will give rise to sensations of light no matter how they are stimulated.

Images falling on the retina after passage through the transparent media of course produce vision. However stimulation of the retina by other routes and stimulation of the remaining visual pathway produce less refined luminescent responses. These stimuli, whether due to trauma, tumour degeneration or vascular imbalance can affect either one eye, or both eyes, or one visual field or both visual fields. However it is a good rule that monocular symptoms mean monocular pathology (Fig. 93).

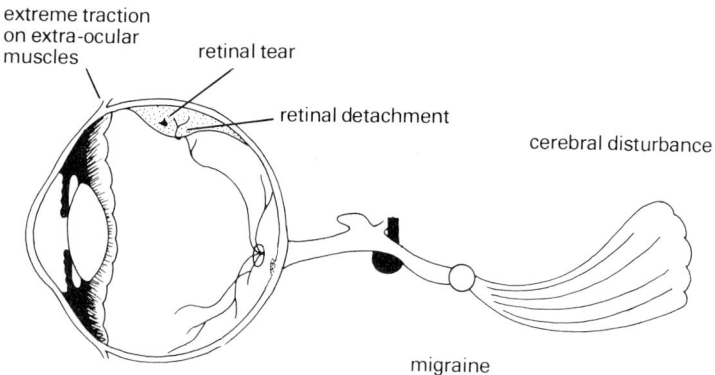

Fig. 93 Flashing lights
Light sensitive tissue in normal or abnormal circumstances can only respond to a stimulus with sensations of light. This clue to the stimulus comes from the type of flash and what other sensations it flashes with

Affections of the eye

Any mechanical disturbance of the retina from within the eye or without can make lights flash. Extremes of gaze can transmit muscular tugging through the sclera to the retina, which in turn transmits these impulses to the brain as transient streaks of light—a premonition of disaster for fanatics who indulge in extra-ocular gymnastics in the interests of health.

Vitreal degeneration
When the vitreous degenerates or collapses its change in position transmits continued impulses to the retina, evident as continued and persistent light flashes. As the vitreous takes up its new position the symptoms may cease after some weeks.

Should the vitreous, however, become adherent to the retina the traction may continue until the retina just gives way. At this point the impulse to light flashing ends in a shower of floaters which announce what has happened. A blood vessel torn at the same time may well add blood to the pigment, and indeed may completely obscure the fundal view.

Trauma
Ocular injuries may result in a silent retinal tear, followed in the long term by a less silent retinal detachment. In the short term, ocular trauma may cause flashing lights, and those of us reared on the *Dandy* comic will recall the galaxy of stars that twinkled in the wake of Desperate Dan's fist. Floaters and subsequent retinal separation were perhaps not subjects calculated to increase the sale of a comic strip.

Pinpoint light flashes in one eye alone must be regarded as serious. A retinal tear must be assumed, until an ophthalmic examination with the binocular indirect ophthalmoscope through the dilated pupil reveals the facts one way or another. Swooping light flashes are not commonly a symptom of impending retinal disaster.

Visual pathways behind the chiasma
The same potential disease processes may affect this part of the system as well.

Migraine
Light flashing from this source is perhaps the most common. Classic migraine, in fact, less common than unclassic migraine, is preceded by a warning aura of flickering scintillating light sensations in one or other visual field. These are considered to be due to the constriction phase of the condition, and in extreme cases may proceed to loss of vision on the affected side—happily not for long.

The vasodilation phase produces the prostrating headache, not usually responsive to standard medications and followed by nausea. Spontaneous onset in tense young people does not indicate the need for neurological examination. In later life, however, it could well be the first sign of some other cerebral disturbance.

Arteriosclerosis and hypertension

Transient variations in the blood flow at random through the cerebral cortex can give rise to casual transient swooping light flashes. Again the age and the general appearance of the patient should indicate which line of limited investigation should be taken.

Temporal lobe tumour

A glioma of the temporal lobe may rarely irritate the visual pathways, and as well as flashing lights, might produce strange phantom figures in the visual field. Commoner irritations of this and other lobes could well explain the sighting of family ghosts in the shadow of an empty decanter of claret.

26

Visual floaters

Any mobile opacity between the retina and the cornea can be called a floater. Most are unimportant, and most people over 30 have these simple floaters anyway. The vital distinction is whether they are of recent origin or not. If they are, they and their associates must also be considered.

Barring the traumatic introduction of foreign material from outside, these floaters must come from the normal ocular tissues. They may be:

1. *Fragments of collagen.*
2. *Blood.*
3. *Inflammatory debris* (Fig. 94).

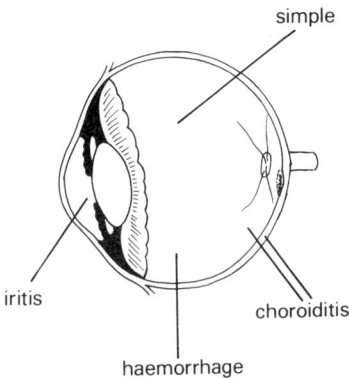

Fig. 94 Floaters
Fresh floaters alone may be significant. Fresh floaters with something else are always significant

Simple floaters (muscae volitantes)

The vitreal cavity is normally full of a viscous structure made up of hyaluronic acid gel that separates slender fibres of connective tissue.

With the passage of time the gel collapses, allowing these normally unseen fibres to coalesce into visibility. They appear in the vision as little wisps and tendrils and tiny circles, most striking against a uniform background of snow or clear blue sky.

That they seem more obvious when we are out of sorts has given rise to the popular belief that they are caused by a 'touch of the liver'. This has led the more austere physicians to believe that a cure can be effected by a total ban on all pleasures. Their more hopeful patients might place more faith in changing the brand name of their pleasures.

Such floaters are recognised by their tenacious return to the centre of vision despite the patient's attempts to shake them away, by their long duration and by a total absence of any other ocular disease.

In certain eyes, usually myopic, such floaters can become coarser still due to further collapse of the vitreous gel. There need be no grave significance attached to their presence.

Gravity and the liquid state of the vitreous necessary for their formation allow them to float downwards out of the line of vision. Sudden activity, however, may shake them upwards at unnerving moments, like a bat threatening the windscreen on a motorway.

Asteroid hyalitis

Just occasionally a casual glance at the fundus in completion of the ophthalmic ritual reveals a glittering suspension of sparkling hard particles holding their position throughout the vitreous and moving with the eye. That their owner is totally unaware of their existence should lead us to be similarly indifferent, for their only significance is what fearful inferences we might draw from their astonishing appearance.

Floaters of sudden and recent onset

Iritis

A scatter of inflammatory cells can dance about in the anterior chamber causing a tantalising degree of visual disturbance. It should be remembered that iritis, the third main cause of the red eye, is the one that may present with no sign other than ciliary injection alone. The presence of floaters in such a red eye may clinch the diagnosis.

Choroiditis

Inflammation in the posterior cavity of the eye is much more rare, and its causes as obscure as those of iritis. There may be little sign of general inflammation, but a hazy vitreous will be seen through the dilated pupil. That nothing else is seen is in itself almost diagnostic.

Vitreal haemorrhage

The bleeding disorders are as likely to present in the eye as anywhere else, they just tend to be more obvious in a transparent organ. Differing as the causes may be, there is nothing particularly diagnostic about the way they affect the eye. They tend to be sudden, with dramatic effusion of opaque debris into the normally clear vitreous. The degree may range from a 'swarm of bees' to total blackness. There are four main causes:

1. *Diabetes.*
2. *General vascular disease (including hypertension).*
3. *Retinal tear and/or retinal detachment.*
4. *Diseases of the blood.*

When contemplated in the abstract, this catalogue might prove as daunting as it does with the patient waiting for an answer and a word of comfort. It need not be daunting if the routine system of examination is coupled with a sharp sense of what is possible and what is likely.

Epilogue

If the whole point of the eye is to see, then the whole point of ophthalmic examination is to keep it seeing. To miss treatable disease is a double tragedy, because with but one small group of exceptions, any condition that might benefit from treatment, even if misdiagnosed at a first attempt, will generally draw attention to itself before it is too late. If the same brief and simple routine of examination be applied every time, then there should not be many episodes of a first time misdiagnosis.

The exceptions are the glaucomas. Closed angle glaucoma, once the angle has closed, will almost diagnose itself. If we are to catch it however while it is still a time bomb, with a narrow yet open angle, a shallow anterior chamber and the odd halo, we need the eclipse test to prevent a preventable calamity.

Glaucoma secondary to recognised ocular disease should be picked up as long as the disease to which it is secondary is still in evidence. However, when that has ceased to attract interest, so may the danger of the secondary glaucoma. At this point it begins to resemble chronic simple glaucoma—by definition secondary to no recognisable ocular disease at all—which may destroy the visual field and all useful vision, unsuspected because no-one has considered the possibility in the first place. To be aware of the possibility is the first step. To look is the second step and to see is to avert the greatest ocular calamity of them all.

However, even before we look at the eye, we must look at and listen to the patient. The revealed history will emerge from what is said, but the concealed history will emerge from how it is said. There is as much again to be deduced from the patient's demeanour: the apprehensive who have nothing wrong but think they have, and the phlegmatic who have everything wrong but think they have not; apoplectic business executives fussing over their bifocals, ageing beauties who refuse to wear bifocals, and pallid diabetics who would settle for any sort of focal.

We can do no better than paraphrase the pronouncement of a

famous detective, celebrated for his curved stem pipe and deer stalker hat, who said that 'when we have eliminated the impossible, whatever remains, however improbable, must be what we are looking for'. He arrived at his conclusions by listening, looking and seeing, and carrying out the same method of investigation every time. His creator was an ophthalmologist.

Index